HEALING SELF, HEALING EARTH

AWAKENING PRESENCE, POWER, AND PASSION

Roy Holman

Holman Health Connections
Everett, Washington

HEALING SELF, HEALING EARTH
AWAKENING PRESENCE, POWER, AND PASSION

Holman Health Connections
1917 Rockefeller Ave., Everett, WA 98201 USA

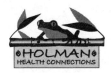

www.holmanhealthconnections.com　　Holmanhealth@gmail.com

All rights reserved. No part of this book may be reproduced or transmitted in any form or by any means, electronic or mechanical, including photocopying, recording, or by any information storage and retrieval system, without written permission from the author, except for the inclusion of brief quotations in a review.

Copyright © 2010 by Roy Holman

Softcover Edition ISBN **978-0-615-29882-5**

First Edition 2010

Book design and illustration:
Linda DeSantis Lapping • DeSantis Design

ACKNOWLEDGMENTS

Ideas and insights from countless people have gone into the creation of this book--too many to acknowledge, but I will mention a few. Thanks to all those who helped with book editing, expertise, and advice: Maggie Bedrosian, Laura Cryan, Bruce Davis, Anita Fieldman, Lee Hart, Linda DeSantis Lapping, Paul McNaughton, Beverly MacCarthaigh, Dena Marie, Gary Perless, and David Seborer. You are angels.

Others played the formal role of teacher, such as my hypnotherapy and spiritual teacher Jamal Rahman, my yoga teacher Tracy Weber, and my hands-on energy teacher Anaiis Salles. Others simply graced me with their daily wisdom, kindness, and compassion: Stella, Louise, Chris, Linda, Pat, David, Jon, Stacy, Barry, Susan, and Brian. Thank you to my family for being brave and putting up with my often-closed heart, and occasional judgments and rough edges. Thanks to my present "family" of housemates: Kay and Devin, and our cats Apple and Mo. I also want to thank all those who pushed my buttons and acted as mirrors for my evolvement. These were perhaps the greatest gifts of all, although it has taken me so many years to understand this.

I once asked our Unity Minister, Robert Eagan, if I could borrow one of his insights from his sermon, and he said, "Of course, everything gets borrowed from the Universe anyway." So, I want to thank the Universe for the inspiration and insights for this book. Thank you, Mother Earth, for your love and patience, and all my tree-friends for your beauty, wisdom, and support.

Special thanks to my good friend Laura, who teaches me how to love.

CONTENTS

INTRODUCTION

This book offers practical and essential tips for living life and being fully human. It is a guidebook for healing and maintaining the body, transforming and integrating the emotions, calming and clearing the mind, and awakening one's deepest spiritual presence.

Ideally, books such as this are unnecessary, in the sense that we all have everything we will ever need. We are whole, nothing is lacking, and we each carry the seed of awakening within us. Books are collections of words, and words cannot easily explain the deepest truth which rests silently in the heart. As you read the following pages, I invite you to remember that we come from wholeness and return to wholeness. We can be devoted seekers, yet not frantic in our quest.

Still, I was spurred to write these words at this time for a reason. These pages may remind and stir you to let go of that which is destructive or shielding your light. For much of my own life, I have struggled with a sense of powerlessness, and often buried both my pain and my passion under a blanket of fear and angst. My hope is that this book will help you to struggle less than I often have, and to create more peace and joy in your life and in our world.

Some of the material presented here was inspired by my many teachers--formal as well as unintentional--while the rest is offered from my personal experience and life lessons. My life brags no famous accomplishments, nor do I have a dozen letters after my name. Yet in all humility, I am doing some of the most essential work on the planet, which few of us--men especially--are taught: looking within, feeling the feelings, entering the shadows, and learning to walk with eyes open and body grounded into the Earth. My journey has taken me through many chapters, including shy Catholic altar boy, hippie-rebel, beer drinking-softball enthusiast, world wanderer; and through diverse careers from butcher, bartender, and carpenter to human rights educator, minister, and my present work as a yoga, meditation, and healing instructor.

The healing encouraged in this book is for each individual self, and also for the benefit of our global community and the Earth

Introduction

itself. The world is only a reflection of what is residing within each of our hearts, and the problems of the outer world are really a manifestation of an inner spiritual and emotional dis-ease. As we feel, heal, and express ourselves, we help heal the Earth. In truth, the Earth is presently healing itself by purifying itself of any harmful energies. This book is therefore relevant, even imperative, for this present moment and this incredible time on planet Earth.

Every generation has its particular challenges, and each moment is unique. We are presently experiencing the end of an estimated 5,125-year cycle, with the current stage of the Mayan calendar concluding on December 21, 2012. Numerous ancient and indigenous peoples, including the Mayans, Hopis, and Sumerians, prophesied an era of great transformation culminating around this very time in which we are now living.

While we may have lost our Selves in many ways, we are awakening, and our world is helping rock and roll us out of our sleep! Our inner worlds are stirring; time itself seems to be accelerating, our very cells vibrating at higher frequencies. While this is an incredibly challenging time on earth, it is a tremendously rich and powerful period in which to be alive. As we individually and collectively rouse ourselves from our delusions, there are some crucial choices to make and the possibilities for transformation are unlimited.

In this book, you may notice that I offer few specific tips for healing our Earth and outer world. I am confident that as our consciousness shifts, our innate, dormant creativity will sprout the specific solutions. My main point in this book is that as we each awaken our presence, power, and passion, bold solutions will naturally and spontaneously arise.

This book is really a workbook for self-healing. Each section is followed by Practice Points and a Contemplation. The Practice Points are suggestions for incorporating the subject into your daily life. The Contemplation is for those who can create a few moments to sit with the topic.

My desire is that the following pages will help reconnect you with your natural breath and compassionate heart. May aliveness be stimulated deep within you, and may feelings and insights arise that stir you to reflect, dance, cry, or laugh. As you read, please invite yourself to be present, breathe easily, and keep a soft gaze and an open heart rather than a hurried or striving mind. Please trust yourself to receive what works and glide past that which does not call you.

My heartfelt hope is that we are each empowered to help create something bold and beautiful. May you be freed to express the greatest gift you can offer our aching yet healing Earth: your Self.

Many blessings on your path, breath by breath.

PRESENCE

To you who suffer,

know this:

Darkness cannot deny

the Dawn.

Pain cannot persist

in your Presence.

Beloved Spirit and Earth

bless and beckon

your truest Power,

your purest Passion,

your Sacred Self.

ROY HOLMAN

PART ONE: PRESENCE

BREATH BY BREATH

We know not what follows: our next breath or our next lifetime.
  - Tibetan saying

Consider giving yourself the gift, right this moment, of one full, natural breath: .... in .... and out .... ah-hhhhhhhhhh. .... How do you feel? Just one conscious breath can bring us back to the present, at home in the body.

Bodies love deep, conscious breathing. It is a gift we can give ourselves anytime, anywhere. We can live without food for many weeks and without water for several days, but we cannot survive without breath for more than a minute or so. We *expire* or die from lack of that which *inspires* us, nourishes us, and sustains us.

Bodies know how to breathe--it is natural and involuntary. We might all die if we had to remember to breathe. We can survive and get through life with short, shallow--often fearful--breaths, but it is our deep, conscious breathing that is emotionally and physically healing. Mindful, natural breathing goes beyond living to thriving, and saying "yes" to life. We are saying: I accept life. I belong here. I have a right to be here.

In yoga, conscious breathing is termed *pranayama*: prana (life or life force) and ayama (to lengthen or regulate). Pranayama

11

refers to the conscious expansion and regulation of the breath, increase of life force energy, and extension of life itself--according to the ancients. When we are aware of the breath, we are connected with the body and the present. Pranayama is transformational, as it re-connects us with the main energy channel, which aligns us with the Divine. Yoga teacher B.K.S. Iyengar says, "Prana is God's breath. Prana is the energy permeating the universe at all levels."[1]

After smoking for 37 years, my mother's final days included chest pain and a breathing machine. On her 85th (and last) birthday, she told me something obvious, "It scares me when I cannot breathe." The reverse is also true: When we are scared, we stop or constrict the breath. There is a strong correlation between breath, thoughts, and emotions. Superficial breathing equals superficial living, afraid of scratching the surface of our feelings.

Most of us are unnaturally shallow and anxious breathers, often disconnected from our body and breath, as well as the present moment. One reason for this is pain. All of us have been frightened or hurt, possibly traumatized or even abused to some degree. Childbirth alone--arriving on planet Earth--can be traumatic! When we are scared or injured, we tend to freeze or contract our breath, and with it our energy. As we do this repeatedly, we create dams of stagnant energies in our body system. Like a river increasingly blocked by debris and branches, these energy blocks stifle the flow of life force through our body. Contracted breath activates the sympathetic nervous system--fight or flight--which tightens the eyes, constricts the body, triggers anxiety, and can even lead to life-threatening illnesses like high blood pressure and heart disease.

When we consider breathing deeply and consciously, we realize that this is no small thing! We are inviting ourselves to free up long-dormant energies, anxieties, and traumas, which means we will inevitably feel them, as they break free or surface. While healing takes us a step outside our comfort zone, we are not seeking to create more pain, but to release the old stuff and make space for more energy, more life!

My yoga teacher, Tracy Weber, says that she sometimes feels apprehension teaching the pranayama aspect of yoga, because invariably some of the students become angry with her. Apparently, as the deep breathing loosens up old wounds, students sometimes project their pain onto the perceived cause of their newly felt emotions, the teacher. Yet, just as fear stops or contracts the breath, the reverse is also true: by courageously and attentively deepening the breath, we activate the parasympathetic nervous system, cleanse the fear, calm the mind, and activate the healing energies.

One of my yoga students, a middle-aged woman named Sandy, told me that she was on an alarming, bumpy flight and began to have a panic attack. Then she recalled what we do in our classes, and took several deep, natural breaths. She was astounded by how quickly her anxiety dissipated and her body relaxed.

Yoga teacher Gary Kraftsow says, "The ancient masters specifically developed the practice of pranayama (regulation of the breath) to balance the emotions, clarify the mental processes, and ultimately to integrate them into one effectively functioning whole."[2] When we breathe deeply, we are saying, "I allow the river to flow; I am not afraid of the current. Although the movement of energy means I will feel life more fully, I know that I can swim in it. I am so much larger, more real, and more powerful than my wounds, for I am the river of life itself. Breath is the wave, washing over me. I am the breath, returning to the sea." As we let the river flow, the muddy emotional waters slowly clear, and we become less angry and moody, more alive and balanced in our energy and emotions.

Following the river of breath leads us to our spiritual Source. In many languages, the word *spirit* and *breath* are interchangeable. One of my yoga students at the local college once asked me: "How do I spiritualize my yoga practice?" This in itself is a wonderful and uncommon question, since yoga in the West is often more about the body than the traditional yogic goals of clearing the mind and union with the Divine. I suggested that she be with the breath; stay connected with it throughout her yoga practice. As we do this in our yoga class, and in our daily lives, we are not only being with the body, but with the movement of spirit in our lives.

Furthermore, we can let the breath (spirit) lead. Just before we react, move, or make any decision, we notice the breath and connect to that which sustains us. This invites spirit to lead our life, and lets the mind and body follow. Breathing deeply and consciously, we respond to life's events rather than react.

Of course, there is nothing wrong with shallow breathing per se. Indeed, during deep meditation one's breath slows, as the churning mind recedes, and a profound, indescribable peace emerges. One's metabolism and heart rate slow--perhaps not unlike a sloth. These meditations can be wonderfully relaxing and joyful. Also, note that *controlled* breathing is actually unnecessary, and releasing control of the breath is a practice in trust and surrender.

Conscious, natural breathing is one simple and powerful practice that can anchor us to the present moment, help us release toxic emotional energy, and calm and clarify the mind. Enjoy and celebrate your breath.

Don't let your throat tighten with fear. Take sips of breath all day and night, before death closes your mouth.[3]
- Rumi

൭ Practice Points

- Throughout your day, simply notice your breath--is it deep or shallow?
- How does the depth of your breath affect your emotional state?
- How does your emotional state affect your breath?
- Notice that when you are aware of the breath, you are present.

Word of Caution: Never strain the breath. Strain not only eliminates the benefits, but is actually dangerous and could provoke serious problems. Pranayama is transformative and powerful, but a qualified teacher is advised.

൭ Contemplation: Breath by Breath

- Observe the natural flow of your breath, in and out through the nostrils, with mouth closed.
- Feel the rise and fall of the chest and belly . . .
- Without strain, begin to slowly extend the length of both the in breath and out breath, easily and comfortably.
- See if there is a natural pause at the end of the in or out breath. Enjoy your breath.

PAY ATTENTION

When you are master of your body, word, and mind, you shall rejoice in perfect serenity.
- Shabkar

The day I sat down at my desk to begin this book, a delicate yellow butterfly landed lightly on my shoulder. My first reaction was to whisk it out the window, quickly set it free, so I could get back to my "work." But then it landed on one of my many stuffed frogs. Now it had my attention, as frogs are my totem friends, and in Native American mythology signify transformation. So I picked up the frog, with the butterfly still holding firm, and placed it gently on my desk, where it joined me for the start of this book.

A couple years later, on the very morning I finished the first draft of this book, I went outside to sit in the grass. Again, a yellow butterfly landed next to me, and we sat together. My little butterfly friends feel like wonderful messengers for this book, helping to give it wings. They also reminded me to take my writing lightly--a challenge for me, as I feel a degree of urgency on Earth at this time. Paying attention--whether to butterflies, our own body, or our Beloved--is one of the main messages in this book.

To be present is to be open to the miracle in each and every instant. Conversely, when we are busy-minded or off traveling away from the body and its precious present, we are not awake to the magnificence in each moment. Presence precedes the peace, power, and passion we seek. We cannot experience and enjoy these rewards without fully showing up--being here now. It's really just that simple.

While being present is simple, it's not so easy. In fact, it sometimes feels humanly impossible, and it may be the hardest thing many of us will ever do. The world calls us outwards, simultaneously in dozens of different directions, away from what is real and life giving.

Yet paying attention makes life so much easier. I cannot tell you how many times I ignored gut feelings, signs, or inner guidance that I should not take a job (it was not for me), write a book (it was not the time), or date a particular person (sometimes we did not make it through the first date). You can save yourself a tremendous amount of time, energy, and money if you learn to pay attention and trust your heart.

Furthermore, paying attention now is an excellent investment for the long term. As we become present and notice what is going on here and now, we naturally come to see what does and does not work as our lives unfold. We become better able to see what helps us move forward, draws loyal friends, attracts fulfilling work, brings in money, or otherwise improves life.

I love that line in the movie *Michael*, in which John Travolta plays the part of a very wise (yet cigarette smoking) angel. Impressed by Michael's insights and intuitive observations, someone asks him how he knows things, to which he quietly replies: "I pay attention."

My friend Pam once told me this sad story: "I was driving down the highway when I noticed two hawks circling over my car, very low. It seemed odd that they were keeping pace with my 50 mph speed, and I remember pointing them out to my passenger and thinking they were trying to get my attention. I then had the thought that they were trying to warn me of something and I should pull over and figure out what their message was. I did not.

"About five minutes later as I was going around a corner, a very clear voice in my head said PULL OFF THE ROAD, NOW! Moments later, an oncoming car swerved into my lane, impossible to avoid, and hit me head on." Pam survived, but not without long-term injuries, which she now views as "souvenirs" to remind her to listen to that inner voice. She gave me permission to use her story, hoping to help others avoid such painful lessons.

There are many ways to learn, but they all require that we show up and pay attention. The healing begins with that attention, as we can only heal that which we become aware of. What is life showing us? We can observe nature's rhythms, notice how animals live, and learn from those humans who live wisely.

Another intuitive friend, Linda, did listen: "I was at a stoplight for a major intersection. The light turned green for me, but something told me to wait. Just then, some young dude came screaming through the intersection at very high speed, running the red light. If I'd gone when the light turned green for me, he could have T-boned us." With attention, we can honor our intuitive, early warning system, and save ourselves from significant pain.

As we pay attention, and as we get honest with ourselves, we notice that we have not been treating each other very kindly. We know something is amiss when we see homeless and hungry brothers and sisters in the streets. We begin to hear the cries of Mother Earth, and we see that we are polluting the waters, fouling the air, and damaging the soil. We notice that it does not feel right to spend over a trillion dollars each year on global military budgets--over half of which is spent by the United States. We notice that short-sighted policies and unsustainable lifestyles are destroying species after species of our fellow creatures. As we pay attention, we notice that our individualistic ideology is depressing us, diverting us into addictions, isolating and separating us from our Selves, and each other.

Yet, as we return our awareness to the heart, we feel compassion. While it is important to notice the pain and problems, it is equally vital that we acknowledge the shift in consciousness, the growth of the environmental movement, the increasing access to varied information and alternative perspectives, and the countless individuals and groups who have risen above their personal concerns to address those of the whole community.

As we pay attention, we notice that instead of giving up, it feels much more nourishing and empowering to be a part of the global awakening.

๑๏ Practice Points

- Stop, from time to time, and notice your external surroundings: sights, sounds, smells.
- Then notice your internal landscape. Am I present? Am I breathing fully? How do I feel?

⚘ Contemplation: Paying Attention

- Without needing to change anything, and without judging yourself, simply notice within: How is my body feeling at this moment? What emotions am I aware of right now? Is my mind calm and focused, or busy and scattered?
- Notice and deepen the breath. Notice the rise and fall of the chest and belly.
- How does the conscious breathing affect the body, mind, and emotions?

COME HOME

Be strong then, and enter into your own body; there you have a solid place for your feet. Think about it carefully! Don't go off somewhere else!
- Kabir

When I was bartending on Cannery Row back in the 1980s, tourists would often ask me how to get to the Monterey Bay Aquarium, just a block away. I would often kid them, "You can't get there from here." In truth, if *there* represents where we want to go--peace, joy, compassion--the *only* way to get there is from *here*.

Coming home to the here and now of the body is not always difficult or complex. In nature, surrounded by beauty and rhythms that are more in tune with one's essential energies, it is easy to be present, at home in one's body, yet connected with the natural world.

Unfortunately, the world most of us live in distracts us, bombards our senses, lures us towards false promises, and makes mockery of our spiritual practice. I once heard a yoga teacher say that if you want to practice presence under the most challenging of circumstances, do it in America. In our urge to make things easy and fun, with all the gadgetry, high tech toys, and material temptations, we have created a culture that urges us in every direction and every time zone except for the here and now--sort of an ongoing jet lag.

Everything happens here, in the present, and the body is always in present time. It is our mind, thoughts, and even spirit that wander. One may ingest *spirits* to feel better, but they are a poor substitute for a missing soul. While it may be fun to ponder the past, plan the future, or move our attention to some tropical beach--and energetically go there--our power is in the present. If we truly want to do what we came here to do, if we want to heal and grow and create a powerful life within our current physical reality, we need to come back to the breath and our earthly home, the body.

The yogis say that someone who is stressed, worried, or anxious has more prana--life-force energy--outside the body than inside. Where the attention goes, our life-force energy and spirit follow. One of the definitions of a yogi is "one whose energy is within their body or space."

Let's consider an analogy. Say you own or rent a house, which represents your body. What happens if you leave your house for a week? The plants get thirsty and perhaps a thin layer of dust settles on the counters. What happens if you leave for a year? There will be a huge pile of mail, more dust, stale air, and dead plants. What if you leave for ten years, with the windows or doors open? Certainly, the home will be a total mess: thieves may have entered, or perhaps people or critters are nesting in your home.

This is essentially what happens when you routinely desert the body. When you constantly let your attention drift away from the present moment, you begin a cycle. More "dust" settles in the body, unaddressed fear and pain accumulate, perhaps even other energies or entities enter, and soon it becomes very hard to get back into your own "house." The lights are off and darkness has descended, and outside is now more inviting than inside. The body has become so crowded with foreign or dense energies that you leave again, where there is more "space," and the cycle continues.

Whether owing to toxic external surroundings and environments, or internal traumas and wounds, many of us have become uncomfortable in our own bodies. Since it is hard to be present in a body with pain, we often create a cycle of leaving the present-- the body--for fantasies of the future or memories of the past. Or, we send our attention or energy off to other places or people--often trying to change *them*! We ourselves become stressed or even sick when we consistently move away from the present moment and our body. Sadly, we deny ourselves the richness of our fully embodied, human experience. More tragically, we may completely lose ourselves in the world.

Coming home to the body and the present, though, may initially feel stressful or uncomfortable, even counterintuitive. Pain may be one of the first things you notice when you become present in your body. You may have initially survived by learning to leave the body, taking your attention away from discomfort *in* the body or perceived danger from *outside* the body. This is not a long-term solution, and eventually creates more pain, as you repeatedly abandon your home, the body.

Rather than criticize ourselves for leaving, however, we can congratulate ourselves every time we come back to the present. As we continue to practice presence, returning "home" over and over again, it does get easier, and being in the body becomes the norm. The pain--or at least the suffering--cannot persist in our consistent and powerful presence.

You begin the process of coming home by noticing when you travel. You pay attention and see how it feels when you leave, and when you are home. When you notice yourself wandering, "spacing out," regretting the past, or fretting about the future, take a deep breath and come home to the here and now.

It is easy to spot people who are home. Their eyes have a spark of aliveness. Drum circles are one example; I love watching people's eyes change as the drumming picks up, just as students brighten during a yoga class. What brings you home? Is it cooking? Singing? Dancing? Gardening? Sitting quietly? Find whatever it is that draws you into the magic of this moment, again and again and again. Create a life and environment that makes it easier to live than to leave.

Come home. This is our profound challenge, simple yet perhaps the hardest and most important thing we will ever do. Your conscious presence naturally and automatically begins the process of dissipating the density, purifying the pain, and relegating the mind to its proper place. Practice makes present.

Don't go outside your house to see the flowers. My friend, don't bother with that excursion. Inside your body there are flowers.[1]
- Kabir

❧ Practice Points

- From time to time, ask yourself: Where am I? Am I in the past, present, or future?
- Is too much of my energy focused externally, maybe trying to force an opinion, gain approval, or control the outcome of a situation?
- What would happen if I smile, bring my attention and energy back to me, here, now? Do I feel safer, more grounded and more powerful?

❧ Contemplation: Come Home

- Take a deep breath, and invite yourself home.
- Just breathe; just be here, now.
- In breath: silently say Come. Out breath: silently say Home.

ARE YOU OUT OF YOUR MIND?

How can you think and hit at the same time?
- Yogi Berra

Are you out of your mind!? Let's hope so. In truth, most of us are very much in our minds, but not the right one!

Zen Buddhism makes a distinction between the "little mind" and the "Big Mind" (or "Buddha Mind," our deepest Self). The little mind makes a great ally, but a bad boss, as evidenced by the madness we see in our world today. The little mind is like a computer in some ways: very handy, holds tons of information, and can organize material; but you would not want your computer making the big decisions, running--or *ruining*--your life.

The little mind is clever and calculating, but not wise. It is creative (as in generating tens of thousands of thoughts a day, many of which create misery), but it is not the source of true creativity and inspiration. The overly busy and ego-centered mind and its programmed memory, like a computer, often contain toxic waste.

Some say mindfulness is a wonderful goal, but I prefer *mindlessness* (even though we associate mindless with trivial pursuits or stupidity). Our minds are already quite full, thank you--less mind might do us all some good. Mindlessness is less mind, and more Mind. With presence, we can make the little mind our ally on our human journey, giving it a role so it can be supportive and helpful. This is the heart of yoga: clarifying and calming the mind. Thus it becomes a wonderful instrument and asset rather than an energy drain or a source of folly.

We need to be patient as we begin to shift attention from the little to the Big Mind. It's like training a cat after she's been accustomed to scratching the couch and carpets. It will take some loving kindness, as well as discipline, to slowly train your mind to come back to the present reality.

Ego and mind are closely related. The ego is built on self and separation, and like the mind, if left unchecked can create havoc in our world. Some say the ego--along with the little mind--must be vanquished, but everything has its place, or it would not exist. Maybe the ego simply provides the experience and illusion of separation for our learning. Perhaps one needs to experience just enough ego for a healthy sense of self, to protect oneself during the human journey. The ego has a place, at least until we awaken enough to dissolve the ego completely, and melt back into the Ocean of One.

When you come back home to the body, the ego will initially resist, but once it gains trust that you are really home and in charge, it will gladly renounce its role. On some level, the ego knows that it is a lousy leader. It is not unlike a teen that may act frustrated when the parents come home, but actually may feel safer, able to surrender the facade of leadership.

The ego and mind also interrelate with our emotions, often pulling us away from the precious present moment. If I have difficulty sleeping one night, it can be an annoyance, but if I begin to worry and think excessively about it, becoming afraid of not being able to sleep in the future ("how will I be able to continue working when I'm tired every day?"), I have turned a small challenge into a nightmare.

In yoga it is often said, "Let the heart lead over the head." We in the West are very developed in the head and mind, but not yet the heart. Our minds are like poorly planned, log-jammed city intersections. We need to re-route some of the traffic of troublesome thoughts and energy through the heart and other energy channels.

A strong intellect can be a protection. I had one student at a yoga retreat who constantly asked questions during class, as if she did not trust her body and self to guide her from the inside out. I suspected that she was staying superficially in the head to avoid pain buried deeply in her body, so one morning I led a breath-connected, meditative class, and invited everyone to remain quiet and trust their body wisdom. This woman honored my request, and during the relaxation time at the end of class I noticed her quietly sobbing. Perhaps she had let herself come out of the head and into the body, where her feelings could be felt and healing could occur.

Remember though, the mind does not have to be an enemy. Naturally and smartly, it seeks to avoid pain and, being a control freak (we give it that control), it likes to project, plan, and manipulate. The mind thinks it needs to do this to avoid suffering and keep a handle on things. It does not have the wisdom to know that only by surrendering to, walking through, or being present with the pain can we journey into the land of freedom.

We can measure our spiritual progress by how much we release reliance on mind, thought, and intellect. As the little mind regains trust in the Big Mind (Being, Soul, our essential nature, or whatever name you call it) showing up in our lives, it may begin to enjoy the relinquishment of all that exhausting responsibility and control. It's a win win win: Good for the mind, good for the Soul, and good for everyone around us. That should put the mind to rest.

ᏮᎥ Practice Points

- From time to time during your day, notice: Who is the boss in this moment? Is it my little mind or Big Mind?

ᏮᎥ Contemplation: Out of the Mind

- Take a few deep, calming breaths.
- Bring your attention into the area above and between the eyes, the place of neutrality (the third eye). Feel presence, neutrality, clarity. Can you feel when you are in the Mind, but not the mind, ego, or thoughts?

- When thoughts do arise, notice without identification or judgment. Let them go without following them. Who is watching?
- After a few minutes, bring your attention down, out of the head, and into the heart. How does this feel?

BECOME EMPTY: SILENCE, SLOWNESS, AND SPACE

I am a hole in the flute that the Christ's breath moves through. Listen to this music.
- Hafiz

I already mentioned the sloth, one of my heroes and teachers because it is by nature the polar opposite of me; I often dart through life like a hungry, bug-eyed goldfish. In 2007, when traveling in Costa Rica during a yoga retreat, our van full of yogis spotted a three-toed sloth on the ground beginning a very slow and dangerous crossing of the highway. It seemed like it didn't have a chance, as speed would be required for success (not being flattened into a sloth pancake). Yet it was its slowness that provided enough time for a local driver to stop, step off his motorbike, and tenderly carry the gentle creature across the road to safety.

There is a retreat center here in Washington state where, upon driving onto the property, a small sign says, "Slow," followed by another further down the driveway that says, "Slower," and then finally a sign advising, "Slowest." These signs always remind us to retreat from the speed and busyness of our normal lives.

Bicycling around Europe taught me that one could see, sense, and experience so much more on a bicycle than in a car. The scenery, people encountered, and wind and sun on the face felt so fresh and real. Walking further slows us down. Then, of course, we can stop. Any pause can provide a wonderful space for grace, gratitude, or guidance to flow into our awareness.

Gandhi said that there is more to life than increasing its speed, and that we must become zero. At one time Gandhi decided to spend one day a week in silence to catch up on all his correspondence, but he also came to find this quiet time as essential to his spiritual renewal. Slowness and silence are not the norm in our busy and noisy world, where decibel levels rise along with the stress level. Contrary to what the world urges, people thrive in slowness and silence, with space to breathe. On an energetic level, spirit and inspiration cannot come into crowded clutter, only into empty space. When we try to cook when busy and hurried, we end up with busy and hurried food.

I found that one of the most valuable things I could do in writing this book was not write. Every six months or so, I would not write, and not read what was already written. Then I could look at it again with fresh eyes. The Koran was delivered to a very patient Muhammad over a period of 23 years. To do this, the Prophet spent considerable time in silence, which provided him the space to receive the powerful guidance.

Stillness can be unnerving to the beginner. At one yoga retreat, we invited participants to eat breakfast in silence--actually only the first ten minutes of the meal. There was one pleasant woman, age 60ish, who was new to yoga, and found the silence very disturbing. Soon she was whispering, "How much longer?" to which Chris, the other teacher, held up an open palm with fingers indicating five more minutes. Two minutes later she rushed over to the whiteboard and wrote, only half jokingly, "HOW MANY MORE MINUTES!??" We all broke into laughter.

Are you carrying too much? There is a story about some travelers who come to a river, and build a raft so they can cross the water. Upon arrival on the other shore, one of them picks up the raft and begins carrying it, until the other reminds her that the raft has served its purpose--she can put it down. Everything has its place, and everything serves a purpose, if we choose to embrace the gifts and lessons. Even our anger, fear, and hate have had a function. But there is also a time to put it down, thank it, bless it, and let it go. We can clear our space.

When we climb a mountain, literally or metaphorically, the closer we get to the peak, the heavier our load feels--and the more important it becomes to lighten the load. Eventually we will need to let it all go so we can reach our final destination--liberation. Are you hauling anything that has become a load, an energy drain, or a burden to you or others? Is there something--a belief, a bitterness, a mistrust in life--you could consider releasing?

In my life, I have been challenged with a belief that I have insufficient money and time in order to take a vacation. During the summer of 2006, I went ahead and took a few days off (after anxiously calculating how much money would be lost), and attended a five-day meditation retreat on Orcas Island, Washington, with the wonderful meditation teachers Joel and Michelle Levy. Even though I've meditated for years, I was amazed at the clarity that filled in the space freed from my mind. The emptiness provided *more* insight, peace, pleasure, and community, and *less* worry, anxiety, and confusion.

The paradox is that emptiness is in truth fullness. One's ego and mind, fearful of losing their jobs, like to fill every moment with thoughts, plans, judgments, and drama. But filling up on junk food appetizers leaves no space for the gourmet main course. It is only by slowing down and clearing space that true intelligence and insight can pour into the emptiness.

Author Lin Yutang says, "If you can spend a perfectly useless afternoon in a perfectly useless manner, you have learned how to live."[1] One of my meditation students recently said that his workmate saw his daily office meditations as weird, until he started joining him. Ever-shrinking vacations have become the custom in the United States, so we have to be willing to step out of the box a bit (or we will prematurely work ourselves into a box in the Earth). Our culture of more work and busyness often results in less joy and being. If all we do is *do*, we have nothing but *do do*!

Chief Seattle said, "There is no quiet place in the white man's cities."[2] (He said this back in the 1850s; what would he think now!?) Perhaps we are afraid of what we may hear in the silence, so every void is filled as if it were a threat. We may fear that if we get quiet, we may have to deal with unfelt emotions and underfed dreams, so we continue filling ourselves with noise and things that may not be comfortable, but are at least familiar.

As you recognize your wholeness, you realize that you have nothing to gain or loose, and this is the essence of liberation. As you surrender the ego's self-importance and illusionary power, competi-

tive attitudes fall away. The desire for external gratification and ob-
session with material things, money, titles, and attention disappear,
leaving a sublime sense of inner freedom and spaciousness.

*When the body empties and stays empty, God fills it with musk and mother-
of-pearl.[3]*
- Rumi

ᏀᏉ Practice Points

- Since ego is one of our major sources of suffering, notice
  whenever you are "full of yourself" and silently say to yourself: less ego, less ego, more Presence, more Presence.
- Periodically throughout the day, consciously make space for
  a releasing breath, or a short break. Consider a nature walk, a
  hot bath, or a nap.
- Clear a space on your calendar for a day off or extended vacation.

ᏀᏉ Contemplation: Hollow Body

- Breathe, and allow your out breath to be one second longer
  than the in breath.
- Imagine your body as hollow, spacious.
- With each out breath, release any of the dense areas, creating
  ever more space for Spirit's breath to flow through you.

KNOW YOURSELF

He who knows himself will know his Lord.
- Hadith

As human beings, we naturally long for a direct experience of who we truly are. Rather than a conceptual understanding
of our deepest nature, we crave the tangible truth of our essential
and everlasting Self. As we discussed earlier, this Big Mind is quite
distinct from our mysteriously changing and evolving smaller self.
It is through the grounded, embodied inner work that we bypass the

ego and come to deeper and more direct contact with who we are. It turns out that we are much more than the ego and mind, for we are the rock, the raindrop, the otter, and the entire cosmos.

When we meet someone, we tend to ask, *What do you do?*, rather than, *Who are you, really? What drives you? What is your passion?* We are often more concerned about our appearance, our resume, or our credit score than the depth of our heart. Our net worth (or debt worth) has become our self worth, and our self-esteem is really dependent on *esteem*--praise, recognition, and acceptance from others.

"I have lost myself."[1] These are the words of Mrs. Auguste D., a German woman of 51 who forgot who she was. In 1907, Dr. Alois Alzheimer reported her to be the first victim of what has become known as Alzheimer's disease. One hundred years later, 13 percent of those over age 65 and nearly half of those over 80 have symptoms of Alzheimer's.[2] Interestingly, regardless of the physiological or biological root causes of Alzheimer's, the disease seems to coincide with an increase in the number of people who have forgotten who they truly are, or what they are here to do. Many of us have become separated from our very reason for being here.

"Who are you?" I give this homework question to my college yoga students. Inevitably, I read answers like: *I am a student, I am a woman, I am a waiter, I am a mother of three, I am angry,* or *I am a Christian.* A mother of nine children wrote: "It is so much easier to answer the question 'what am I?' than 'who am I?'" Yet what we are is temporary, whereas who we are is permanent. We also ask this same question as a wonderful, although initially uncomfortable, exercise in our workshops. We pair up, decide who goes first, and then repeatedly ask the person, "Who are you?" hearing their answer each time. Initially, the response is as above, but eventually, the superficial layers peel away, and the deeper realization--often accompanied by tears--emerges.

It is impossible to suffer from self hate when we really get to know our deepest, most beautiful Self. In the *Bhagavad Gita*, Krishna tells Arjuna, "But ignorance is destroyed by knowledge of the Self within."[3] One way to know the Self is by getting to know the self, or that which we are not (ego, mind, feelings, beliefs, castes, titles). We are not who we *think* we are. As we release identification with temporal personality, there is a reconnection with Self.

Yet we are wise to get to know our feelings, as they are trustworthy guides. Feelings offer a bodily response to what the Spirit is doing, and they provide communication and feedback to the Spirit as to bodily needs and desires. In touch, but not attached to your feelings, you can freely be your whole, connected self, and are better able to help others liberate themselves from the trappings of their own limitations and dramas.

Our Western world tends to identify with the ego, with its emphasis on selfishness and superiority. We glorify and make heroes out of highly-paid sports stars and other celebrities, regardless of their contribution to the whole. One may have an impressive knowledge of sports statistics and other irrelevant information but know little of one's body, mind, or Soul.

While sacred service requires a commitment to both the inner and outer work, at times your service work may be simply getting to know yourself. When you are hurt or hurting, this may be a time for retreating, receiving, and getting to know who you really are. This is what I had to do after my human rights work in Guatemala, when it became obvious that I needed to pull back and deal with my own issues, lick my wounds, and acknowledge my motivations. It turned out that a good part of what I thought was selfless service was actually ego- and wound-driven, diverting my focus away from my own inner pain.

The ancients in their teachings have invited us over and over to "know thyself." Jesus said, "Deny yourself," which means releasing the over-identification with the body, mind, ego, and drama. But how do you get to know your true Self? You might begin by admitting you do not know, humbly realizing that you are lost. Let your daily intention be one of self-discovery. Then pay attention.

Yoga is one time-tested tool for self-knowing. The Yoga Sutras (ancient writings on yoga) speak of two kinds of knowledge. One comes through inference and observation, such as studying sacred texts, while another arrives through intuition and direct inner experience. A measure of quietude is required to "simply know." "Yoga" means "to yoke," or unite, referring to the integration of body, mind, and Spirit. As we continue to grow spiritually, we come to know the mind and body as wonderful but transient aspects of our human experience.

At the end of each yoga class, we say to each other, "Namaste," which means, "The Divine in me bows to the Divine in you." Imagine a world where people see and honor the Divine in themselves and in one another. War would end, and peace would reign.

As we feel and come to know Oneness, our identity with the totality, we are free. When we know that no one is better than anyone else, we are seeing clearly. When the voice of God feels like our own inner voice, we know God and we know our Selves, for they are One.

A sense of separation from God is the only lack you really need correct.[4]
- A Course in Miracles

⊙ **Practice Points**
* Throughout the day, begin to notice when you identify with your job, title, salary, or body.
* Ask yourself, "Who am I really?"

⊙ **Contemplation: Who Am I?**
* Breathe and relax your body.
* Ask yourself: Who am I? First allow yourself to feel the question, and then answer from the heart.
* Who am I? Who am I? Who am I?

LOOK WITHIN

If I do not go within, I go without.
- Neale Donald Walsch

What do preachers, teachers, political pundits, investment analysts, and meteorologists all have in common? They are often wrong but we generally trust them. Many of us have come to believe that outside authority figures have more information, more intelligence, or have better connections--perhaps to God--than ourselves.

The images and messages incessantly conveyed through the media also reinforce the notion that happiness and information lie outside ourself. The commercials, songs, and movies demonstrate that we are incomplete without that partner, car, beer, credit card, or latest gizmo. We may look and search more deeply into the refrigerator than our own heart and mind.

Despite the obvious Earthly pleasures--a fulfilling relationship, a magnificent sunrise, or fragrant flower--it is ourselves and our deepest connection with the universe that we truly seek. The yoga sutras say, "For those who seek liberation wholeheartedly, realization is near."[1] We only need to recognize and embrace what is already here, right now.

Increasingly, I have yoga students who have been advised by their doctors to try yoga. These students often arrive with specific instructions about what they can and cannot do, and of course, doctor's orders must be honored; they generally make sense. Isn't it sad, though, that so many of us depend on someone else to take care of our own body? We currently spend more on healthcare than any other country, yet we have less wellness than many industrialized (and even some undeveloped) nations. Health care practitioners are vital, but we can pay attention, trust ourselves, and learn to take more personal responsibility.

There has been an increase in the number of yoga injuries in the U.S. In part, this is due to the increasing number of people doing yoga, but I wonder if there is another reason. Our Western world is heavily imbalanced towards the yang (more "do and push" oriented than "be and allow"). At the same time, we are often a bit ungrounded, disconnected, and busy. This combination is hazardous to our health! Yoga is an ideal remedy because it helps us center and reconnect with the body. Still, until we are reconnected enough to understand the body's needs and limits, we may follow the teacher's ideas over our own, push too hard, and sometimes hurt ourselves.

Yoga teaches us to pay attention; our presence and awareness penetrate every part of the body and energy system. When we are connected to the breath, body, and inner voice, we hurt ourselves less, and grow and heal a lot more. Clearing the mind and awakening our deepest truth are the real goals of yoga.

I have always had a tough time looking within and trusting myself with decisions. Even the simplest decision would cause me deep and prolonged anxiety. Whether deciding which movie to see, or what job to apply for, an agonizing sense of despair would overcome me. Even now, I sometimes find it difficult to access my inner wisdom, and I trust other's opinions over my own. Still, I am learning. Countless times when my mind was troubled I have sat in stillness, breathed deeply, and within minutes would receive an answer, a shift, or a profound feeling of peace. *A Course in Miracles* tells us, "Peace is an attribute in you. You cannot find it outside."[2]

Here is a specific personal example. One day, my friend Laura and I were driving up the highway, when something triggered me and I became distant and defensive. After a few very uncomfortable moments, I asked her to excuse me for a moment and closed my eyes (she was driving!). Within moments the memories, fear, and pain at the core of my reaction dropped away--along with a few tears. Just like that, I touched base with what was real and alive in that moment. I apologized and shared with Laura what was up, and the rest of the day was a joy.

Sitting in stillness and looking within do take courage. We are not taught this in school! One of my college students wrote on her homework: "There are those times when it simply hurts too much to look inside." The inner work is the path where only the brave--or perhaps the desperate--venture. What we find is so worth the search.

Heaven is within. Wisdom, joy, and true intelligence arise from the depths of Self, that profound pool of creativity that has access to our biggest--and smallest--questions. Tune in to it. Trust it. For it is You.

✺ Practice Points

- At times, when you consider advice or instructions from others, take a deep breath and ask yourself: Does this sound correct? Do I already know my answer? What is my truth?

⊚ Contemplation: Going Within

- Breathe deeply, and let yourself settle beneath the clouds of consciousness, beyond the thoughts and emotions.
- Allow a sense of stillness or peace to emerge from the silence, and just be with this. Access the place that knows.
- If you feel called, formulate a question and, without effort or expectations, be open to feelings, words, or images that may represent an answer.

BEING YOU: TRUTH AND AUTHENTICITY

To thine own self be true.
  - Shakespeare

Be yourself. Just be yourself. Sounds simple enough, doesn't it? Once we learn how to come home, go within, and know ourselves, all we need is to be ourselves.

Well, maybe this is not so easy. Does the thought of being yourself, speaking your truth, and expressing your passion stir feelings of confusion or frustration? Does it bring up fear or anger? Were there times in your life when you tried to just be yourself and it wasn't really appreciated? Maybe you tried to be loving, or honest, or express an emotion and it was not well received. Perhaps you were invalidated, or even shamed. Maybe you were taught that being yourself was simply not enough, that you had to be special, better, or "perfect" before you were acceptable.

For much of my life, I have been haunted by the terrifying belief that being myself was not nearly enough. Having had few healthy role models in my childhood, and knowing little about who I truly was, I readily followed anyone who appeared to know what they were doing or talking about. At age 19, I worked with a big, loud fellow, about ten years older than myself, who seemed so powerful, cool, and confident. How I longed to be less shy, more self-assured like him! Later, his marriage and life fell apart, and it became clear that he was very insecure, with big masks and arrogance covering up his deep insecurities.

A local beauty salon has a sign in the window, Be Beautiful. Be Yourself. Below the words is a photo of a glamorous fashion model. But does an expensive hairstyle make someone more oneself? Does the cover of the book really foretell its essence? Our culture confuses the exterior with the interior, often at a painful price. Like the Velveteen Rabbit from the children's storybook, there is a time to get real, to recognize and reveal the essence beneath the shell.

Are you being yourself? If not, who are you being? Are you being your authentic Self, or your egoist self? Are you being the beautiful (regardless of your hairstyle) and powerful person you came here to be, who God or the Universe created? When you speak, do you hear your own voice of truth and power? If not, whose voice do you hear?

Or, do you create so much busyness that there is no time for what matters, what brings you joy, being real and true to your Self? Are you too wrapped up in the human drama, acting like someone else? The world needs you to show up in the fullness and greatness of who you are.

Many of us learned early on that being ourselves was not enough, or not okay. *Who are you to be so bright or bold?* Those parents and adults who, as children, were not given a safe space to be their own full, magnificent selves unconsciously limit the authenticity in others. We do what we were taught.

It may have been dangerous to be ourselves. Jesus, Joan of Arc, Gandhi, Martin Luther King, Jr., Nelson Mandela, and Aung San Suu Kyi (Burma's imprisoned leader who won the Nobel Peace Prize in 1991) are exceptional examples of people who spoke their truth. They were their powerful authentic selves, and of course, they were killed or imprisoned for it. Many of us fear, even as we envy, those who demonstrate what we ourselves are afraid to say or do.

Paramhansa Yogananda said, "The Hindu scriptures declare that those who habitually speak the truth develop the power of materializing their words. What commands they utter from the heart will come true in life."[1] We can practice authenticity in words, action, and even thoughts. Honesty heals, and what we put out into the world comes back around to us. Hurtful acts and dishonest deeds cannot result in loving, healing outcomes. Yet one true statement can dissipate dozens of deceits.

The Yoga Sutras use the Sanskrit words *satya* (truth), and *ahimsa* (nonviolence), which Gandhi combined and utilized in transforming India. We need to align our truth with the compassion of the heart. If we are not careful, honesty can be thinly disguised hate, jealousy, or cruelty. There is an Arabian proverb: "When you shoot an arrow of truth, dip its point in honey."

To heal, we first need to become real, willing to recognize and open up the wounds, which at first may feel counterintuitive and countercultural. There is an Ethiopian proverb, "He who conceals his disease cannot be cured." Do not let pride mask your wounds. When you are strong enough to be vulnerable, and reveal your soft side, you may find that the world, rather than tear into your underbelly, may offer a healing touch and help guide you back to yourself.

When we are open and truthful with others and ourselves, we say to the universe and prove to others that we are trustworthy. We begin to attract more sincere and reliable people into our lives. Living an authentic life means giving permission not only to yourself, but also to others to be true to dreams, heart, and gut.

Gandhi said that the ends must match the means. He used the word *satyagraha*, literally meaning "holding onto truth" or "soul force." We are presently moving into a new paradigm, where satyagraha is essential.

And you will know the truth, and the truth will make you free.[2]
- Jesus, in John 8:32

ᇰᅠ Practice Points
- In your daily interactions with people, notice how it feels when you are being authentic and genuine, versus fearful or phony.
- How does it feel when you tell the truth? How does it feel to your body? To your Soul?

ᇰᅠ Contemplation: True to Self
- Give thanks and have compassion for your masks, yet let them soften and peel away.

- Breathe in: I am honest and authentic with myself.
- Breathe out: I am honest and authentic with others.

MEDITATION AND PRAYER

Be still, and know that I am God.
- Jesus, in Psalm 46:10

In 1905, Albert Einstein was reportedly staring out the window and daydreaming when he had the insight that evolved into the Special Theory of Relativity.[1] It has already been mentioned how wisdom and guidance cannot come into--or out of--a busy body and messy mind. Silence is sacred, and Spirit lays waiting in the stillness.

As with anything, let's not get attached to labels or "shoulds," including meditation and prayer. There are walking, sitting, and many other forms of meditation, and there are many ways to pray, reflect, and find solitude. Although many of our activities--even yoga or gardening--can be more doing than being, some of us need to move the body in order to calm the mind or feel Divinity. Who says we cannot gain clarity or find our God while swimming or knitting? Sometimes the mind may be too busy to sit in meditation or prayer, and you may get more calm and clarity walking in the forest, where the energy is clear.

Certainly meditation is about *being* more than *doing*, and many activities are simply too active to help us access that deepest peace. Even in meditation, the ego can easily trick us into doing, in its myriad of subtle and not so subtle forms: searching for answers, wanting clarity, needing a certain result, or attaching to enlightenment, in effect transforming our meditation into a mind-and-goal-oriented thinking session.

I love both teaching meditation and actually sitting in meditation and prayer. It has taken me some years to get comfortable with it, but I now look forward so gratefully to my morning sitting; I cannot begin to tell you what a difference this has made in my life. Simply put, meditation slows me down, but it also provides a daily space for praying, counting blessings, and voicing and visualizing intentions. Sometimes, a quiet reassurance is felt, or answers to questions. At times, I get in touch with buried emotions, with their sometimes uncomfortable yet liberating energies or tears. Or, I make contact with the Everything, an energy that feels like the Spirit of my heart. Sometimes old patterns shift, and new paths emerge from the richness of silence.

Of course, my meditations are sometimes one big frustration, where I just sit and watch the mind run laps around my head-- and this is okay too. Yet difficult work can bring great rewards. The demons of mind chatter, critical voices, and attachments soften or disappear when we face them directly and invite their integration.

There are many styles of meditation: mindfulness, insight, Zen, Tibetan and other Buddhist styles, mantra (sacred sound), and Christian contemplative prayer, to name a few. I call the style I do and teach Integrative Meditation, since I incorporate the techniques and tools from numerous traditions to fit what is needed. Trust yourself to experiment and do what works. Whatever style of meditation you choose, I highly recommend you find one that brings you fully into the body. Along with compassion, this is the most important and beneficial key to transformative meditation: being embodied and feeling deeply into the emotions and sensations of the body. We find enlightenment through--not away from--the body.

Some say that prayer is talking to and honoring God, and meditation is listening. Some of us choose to combine prayer with meditation, as prayer is a profoundly reassuring practice that re-unites us with our Beloved. It can be counting blessings, or simply reminding ourselves of what is real and important. Muslims often say, "One prostration to God frees you from a thousand prostrations to your ego." Desire for our Beloved may be the only desire we need. *The Bhagavad Gita* claims that the path of devotion is one of the surest ways to freedom. Passionate devotion moves us out of the ego and adds a key element of emotion to our longing, accelerating our inner journey.

Thinking during meditation will not ruin it, unless you think so! When you have a thought, think nothing of it, for the mind's job is to think. Simply choose something else; bypass the mind and go deeper. There is a tremendous and profound difference between thinking, and the clear awareness of our Being. Thinking has its place, and most meditations have elements of both thinking and being. Yet at our core lies true wisdom, creativity, and lucidity, which arises from beyond the thinking mind. This is the realm of spirit, miracles, and limitless inspiration. As it is not a place, we cannot get there; we can only be there. We can be there--or here--not by doing, although we can set the stage for it by making time, being quiet.

Before we can just be there, we may need to calm the body with yoga, or wake up with a morning shower. For some, creating a sacred space for meditation can help. Although Spirit requests a hefty payment--releasing attachment to ego--our Beloved is also a cheap date, needing no incense, candles, exotic music, or special decor. If these help, use them. A space that feels safe and healing can be helpful, however that looks to you. Rest assured, though, that the Divine requires no fluff--only an open and willing heart.

Beginner's mind is a Zen Buddhist term for sitting with openness and without expectations and preconditions. Beginner's mind is often our greatest asset for meditation training, which may go something like this: beginning meditation class, then intermediate meditation class, then advanced class--where you ideally forget all the fancy techniques you learned in the first two classes! Then we can get back to basics and "beginner's mind," which is an effortless, embodied yet expansive presence.

Meditation is sometimes defined simply as nonjudgmental awareness, or presence. While our goal may be to calm the mind, find our true path, or awaken to our deepest nature, another way of approaching this is "no goal." Our "goal" is simply to be. According to the Yoga Sutras, since it is hard to move from many thoughts to no thoughts--busy mind to empty mind--we start by withdrawing our sense inwards (pratyahara), then follow this with concentration (dharana), and then ideally move into ever more empty, effortless being (dhyana or samadhi). Concentrating on and connecting with the breath is an excellent anchor.

Be present. Be the silent witness. Release thoughts and pay attention to what arises: sensations, emotions, insights, and so on.

Have compassion for all of it. That is all.

Meditation is one of the simplest, yet most challenging things we can do. Since most of us have very undisciplined minds, please do not punish yourself if you cannot sit still. Have compassion, which itself is a wonderful focus for meditation. Start with a few minutes a day, or whatever works for you. If you think you don't have time for meditation and prayer, think again. Better yet, move beyond thought.

Stop the words now. Open the window in the center of your chest, and let the spirits fly in and out.[2]
- Rumi

Practice Points

- Consider making your very life a meditation or prayer, being present and prayerful whenever possible.

Contemplation: Breath of Compassion

- Sit quietly, and breathe easily. Imagine roots grounding your body down into the Earth, like an old-growth tree.
- For a few minutes, extend the breath longer and deeper, without strain. Allow the out breath to be one second longer than the in breath, and if comfortable, allow a natural pause at the end of the out breath--perhaps a second--before your next in breath.
- Let the goal of this meditation be to have compassion for yourself. When any thoughts or emotions arise, feel compassion, silently smile, and come back to the breath.
- Be more than do. Accept rather than judge. Breathe compassion.

PART TWO: BODY AND EMOTIONS

LOVE AND MOVE YOUR BODY

If it weren't for the fact that the TV set and the refrigerator are so far apart, some of us wouldn't get any exercise at all.
- Comedian Joey Adams

Your beloved body wants nothing more than to be loved. Like trying to drive an old broken down car or bicycle, it can be frustratingly difficult for a soul to work through a body that is unhealthy or uncared for.

Of course, much of our Western world is preoccupied with the body. Yet cosmetic surgery and ten thousand dollar makeovers are not necessarily signs of genuine care for the soul's cathedral, but often signs of insecurity and misguided values and perceptions. Often, we are incapable of seeing and appreciating our innate beauty, so the body is excessively adorned or altered.

Even as we fuss over our physical appearance, many of us are disconnected from the body. While many body-focused people ignore spirit, many spirit-minded people ignore the body. We may even attempt, perhaps unconsciously, to "ascend" prematurely to heaven or into the spirit world by withdrawing our energy from the body and the Earth up into the head or even out of the body. We abandon our own body. This describes me for much of my life, where being human felt like too much pain and work. Looking back,

I now see that I often spaced out, or withdrew energetically from the body, which held tremendous emotional pain.

But are we not here, in body, on Earth, for a reason? Furthermore, if we were not supposed to enjoy these earthly and bodily delights--eating, sunshine, lovemaking, swimming, and so on--they would not *feel* so good. When you do not trust and honor your body and allow it, with discernment, pleasure and movement, you grow bitter, miserable, and lifeless.

This view is the Middle Way discussed in Buddhism and by Jesus, "in the world but not of it." In the later stages of their lives, the Buddha, St. Francis de Assisi, and other sages reportedly warned against excessive fasting and other extremes of spiritual austerities. This middle path includes being vigilant and honest in order to avoid both excess piety as well as gluttony.

The great, devoted yogi Paramhansa Yogananda said, "The consciousness of a perfected yogi is effortlessly identified, not with a narrow body, but with the universal structure."[1] While this is so true and essential, we must be careful here. It is all sacred: the Body, Bones, Blood, and Being. We who are spiritually focused can stop judging and resisting our humanity and learn to fully embrace this human adventure. As angelic and alluring the afterlife may seem to us, we had best keep our attention and awareness here in the body, feeling or finding the heaven within. It is exceedingly difficult to bring conscious presence into a body you belittle, as wise teachers like Yogananda were well aware of.

At a recent workshop, I guided the participants in a meditation on our relationship with food, inviting each person to listen to the body's messages. In the discussion afterwards, one woman, clearly triggered by the meditation, remarked, "It doesn't matter what we eat." Perhaps not coincidentally, she appeared overweight, which is an epidemic in our country. Although she was an accomplished author and spiritual teacher, at this point she may have been unwilling or unable to truly hear or honor her body. Again, some of us are spiritually focused, yet physically denying or disconnected.

Not only is the body the temple for Spirit, the body itself is a manifestation of the Divine. To create a body, or any manifestation in the world of form, the "fast vibration" energy of spirit is slowed down, condensed into the world of form or matter. Still, it is all energy, and without life force and spirit's presence pulsing through it, the body withers into sluggishness and decay.

At times, we may give the body everything it demands, and life becomes a hedonistic funfest. At other times, the pendulum swings back and we become self-punishing, perhaps excessively dieting or depriving ourselves. My personal pendulum has swung dramatically, between fast foods and fasting, from godlessness to god-based cults. When you bounce from pleasure-seeking to monastic frugality, you are ignoring the genuine needs and innate wisdom of the body, which seeks balance. You can be present, loosen the control, and trust the body.

Perhaps everything has its place. Some of us may even choose to meditate in a cave for ten years; if that is your path, great. At some point, though, you have to leave the cave. Some of us may be pure love in meditation or in our spiritual group, yet short-tempered grumps when someone cuts us off in traffic (often, that's me). We may be peaceful by ourselves but sloppy in relationships. You can invite yourself off the cushion or couch, move the body, and connect with this world. That's why they call it a spiritual practice.

Your body is a miracle! It is a magnificent creation--God's creation--and it houses the miracle of you. It has simple needs: When tired, rest. When hungry, eat. When thirsty, drink. When stiff, move. Giving the body what it truly wants and needs is not difficult, if you are present, tuned in, ever alert to the temptations of the world.

Bodies thrive on activity and play. Like rivers, bodies need to move and flow. There is a deeply satisfying and fully embodied joy in dancing, drumming, or simply stretching or walking. The people I most easily relate to are the ones most presently alive and whole, fully celebrating their humanity, not busy planning their spiritual afterlife or next incarnation!

I know one accomplished naturopath and healer who tells her patients that the first thing to do to improve their health is choose some sort of exercise or movement that pleases them and their bodies. Whether it is hiking or hockey, badminton or basketball, let the body do what it loves to do, or it will rebel. Among its many benefits, exercise relieves depression, lowers weight, improves glucose utilization, helps us sleep better, and raises self-esteem.

Bodies also need to touch and be touched. In an era of voice recognition software, internet communication, and lawsuits over inappropriate touching in the workplace, many people have become further isolated and afraid of safe and compassionate hugs and touches. Enjoy every opportunity to feel: the shampoo in your hair, a cool breeze in your face, the stone in your hand, your bare feet on the earth.

There is a wonderful balance to be found between forced asceticism and unconscious overindulgence of the body. Embody Spirit, for pleasures of the flesh will never be complete without true Presence. Yet know that the body is deeply intelligent as well. When you truly inhabit, honor, and trust the body, it finds balance, for it knows exactly what it needs.

Spirit and body make excellent dance partners, but neither should dominate or ignore the needs of the other. Spirit and body-- enjoy the dance.

∿ Practice Points

- When you first wake up in the morning, what does your body need? A glass of water? Shower? Foot massage? Take a moment to do so.
- Pay attention to your body throughout the day. If you can't make time for a yoga class or a walk, can you stretch, or simply take a deep breath?

∿ Contemplation: In the Body

- Breathe deeply, and notice: the miracle of your body.
- In breath: Notice the rise of the chest, and opening of the heart.
- Out breath: lowering and relaxing of the belly and navel.
- Ask your body: What healthful kind of food, movement, or activity do you love but not get enough of? Honor what you hear, and discern what is appropriate.

YOGAAAHHHHHHHHH . . .

Arjuna, cut through this doubt in your own heart with the sword of spiritual wisdom. Arise; take up the path of yoga!
- Krishna, in Bhagavad Gita

I began yoga in 1995, and have found no better way to love, connect with, and move my body. I had just turned forty, and was struggling with depression, an eating disorder, and mid-life issues. Walking out of that first class was a revelation. Despite all my pain and confusion, I felt grounded, refreshed, and renewed. I've now been teaching yoga and meditation for over ten years, and I have come to see that it is beneficial for most anyone, and especially for our disconnected, anxious, and mind-oriented Western world.

Yoga is a multi-dimensional healing art and science that includes poses, conscious breathing, meditation, and lifestyle choices to bring balance, strength, and flexibility on the physical level, calm and centering on the mental level, healing and integration at the emotional level, and Self-awareness and awakening on the spiritual level. The overall goal and reward is enhanced health, aliveness, and connection in body, mind, and spirit.

While teaching yoga at the community college, I came to notice that my younger students were having a tough time being fully present for the early morning classes. Like many of our youth, they were often tired, stressed, and over-stimulated, and it was challenging to keep their attention for the few minutes of "lecture" prior to the yoga poses; their eyes glazed over and they spaced out. Then one day I did an experiment: we did the yoga poses and breathing *before* the heady part of the class. What an amazing difference! After just a short yoga practice, they were incredibly present, bright-eyed, and attentive for the cognitive part of the class. It validated how yoga can bring us home.

It is one thing to say, "Be present," but another to get there, or even understand what this means. Yoga systematically and safely alters the particular energetic state of the individual to create the optimal conditions for being present. Yoga is an invitation into the body and the present moment, where all healing and growth occur.

Ultimately, yoga is about clearing the stagnation in the body and mind enough to wake up to our true essential nature. Yoga poses *(asana)* and breath work *(pranayama)* cleanse the body and mind and prepare us for meditation, where we may get a sense of our greater Self. We begin to relate more from that calm, clear core.

Yoga, in one form or another, is for everyone. If you can breathe, you can do yoga (if you can't breathe, well, that's called corpse pose!). In the West, yoga is often more of an exercise routine, and many people do it for purely physical reasons, to stretch, strengthen, or balance, or even to look sexy or spiritual. That is fine, but yoga is so much more than asana, six pack abs, and long hamstrings. People often begin yoga for one reason and stick with it for more profound benefits: reduced anxiety, better focus, more aliveness, and a greater sense of self and purpose. One of my male students remarked, "I find that as my body gets stretched, so does my mind. I feel calm and clear."

More than exercise; yoga is really energy medicine. The key to a strong yoga practice is not the strength of the pose, but the connection to the breath. When we connect the movement to the breath, magic happens, or perhaps more accurately, presence happens. We increase the flow of life force and move the *prana* or *chi* through the body. As we connect the body, mind, emotions, and spirit, we become present and fully embodied.

Another powerful aspect of yoga is chant and the use of sound. The ancients understood that vibration has a profoundly transformative and healing effect on emotional wounds and energetic blockages. Furthermore, chanting and *kirtan*--call and response chanting--are time-tested remedies for poor memory and busy-mindedness. As Gina Salá, a wonderful chant leader and voice teacher in Seattle says, "When I try to meditate, oftentimes it's monkey mind, but chanting quickly and immediately gathers my focus in a delicious way and brings me home." Chanting has been little used in the West--although Native peoples have used it for millennia--and is sometimes beyond people's comfort zone, as we have so many wounds around using our voice. In recent years, though, its benefits and heart-expanding joy is catching on, with people like Krishna Das, Deva Premal, and Snatam Kaur Khalsa leading kirtans in packed houses. Try it, if you feel called.

Although it originated in India, yoga works independent of any religion or spiritual philosophy. It may help you clarify your beliefs and perhaps deepen your practice, whatever it is, or it may spur you to leave all beliefs and attachments behind. I had one student tell me that her friend wanted to come to class but could not because she was a Christian! I was sad that due to an erroneous belief, she was missing the opportunity to do yoga. Yoga is not Hindu, Buddhist, nor Christian, and it is any or all of these. Yoga is about discovering your own way Home.

If you are at all called to try yoga, I recommend you experiment with different teachers and styles, as there is a huge range out there. Trust yourself. Some teachers or styles will cause you to run for the door, while others may feel like one big ahhhhhhhhh! Bypass the ouch and look for the ah! Yes, progress requires discipline, commitment, and stretching your edge, but pain is not necessary for gain.

If yoga still does not feel right, then by all means consider Tai Chi, Qigong, or whatever clears, grounds, and quiets your body and mind. But, make sure it is something that attracts you to your center, rather than distracts you from your Self.

Yoga, through which divinity is found within, is doubtless the highest road. But discovering the Lord within, we soon perceive Him without.[1]
- Ram Gopal

꧁ Practice Points

- Try this simple yoga movement, sitting or standing: Breathe in while you slowly reach your arms out to the side and up overhead . . . exhale as you slowly lower your arms to your side.
- Gradually lengthen the breath without strain, moving the arms ever more slowly: in breath up, out breath down . . . several rounds.
- Allow and feel an integration of body, mind, and spirit.
- If you feel called, try a local yoga class.

ஒ **Contemplation: Simple Yoga**

- Sit comfortably, deepening the breath.
- On in breath, feel expansion of upper chest, solar plexus, and belly.
- On out breath, feel chest and belly drop, actively drawing navel inwards.
- Also, on every in breath, elongate the spine by lifting top of head slightly.

FOOD AND NUTRITION

If man made it, don't eat it.
  - Jack LaLane

When we do yoga and other healthful practices and disciplines that connect us with our body, we eventually stop obsessing over diets and rules around eating. As we become more attentive and alive in our body, we instinctively know how to care for it and what to eat.

A study of 15,500 middle-aged men and women at Fred Hutchinson Cancer Research Center found that those who practiced yoga regularly did not gain weight in middle age like most people.[1] It's not that the yoga practice necessarily resulted in sweating or burning off the calories, but rather, unhealthy habits seemed to fall away as people become more conscious and focused on eating and living more healthfully.

Eating right is both simple and complex. It is natural to give the body what it needs, but it seems confusing and challenging because we have gotten into our heads and lost touch with the body. The reason we need rules and diets is that we have forgotten how to listen to our bodies, which are always whispering--and sometimes shouting--their needs and preferences. Yoga helps us listen.

I believe that most of us in the United States have patterns of disordered eating, and few of us have wonderful relationships with food and our bodies. How many of us eat exactly what we need, only when we are hungry, and just the amount to satisfy our body's nutritional needs of the moment?

Increasingly, many areas of our world suffer from food shortages, or distribution and sharing problems, making it a luxury to eat. Still, many of us are blessed with an abundance of foods of all flavors, along with nutritional information. The road to healthful eating is no mystery, yet so many of us who do have access to healthy foods still eat junky, depleted, or denatured foods, and two thirds of Americans are overweight or obese.

Our government has not always been as influential as corporate advertisers have: In 2008, for every dollar the USDA spent on nutritional education, the food industry spent $24 on ads and marketing to sell their products, which are not always all that healthful.[2] We can take responsibility for ourselves. Suing a fast food corporation for making us fat may not be the only solution. We can reconnect, re-educate, and re-empower ourselves.

Personally, I tend towards organically-grown, nutrient rich foods: dark green vegetables, whole grains, raw nuts, avocadoes, tofu, chicken, and fresh fruits. I also enjoy sea veggies, which are packed with minerals. Wheat--especially refined wheat--does not work for me, and I do not like the smell or taste of most microwaved food. I drink purified or spring water, and I try to carry my water in stainless steel or glass when possible, as most plastic does not taste right and reportedly leaches toxins into the water. I also enjoy green and herbal teas. Alcohol feels less and less acceptable to my body.

Many of us have an unreasonable fear of fats. Healthy fats and proteins are necessary, especially with breakfast, but ideally all through the day. Healthy fats will not fatten us. Americans began gaining weight when we became more sedentary, increased our intake of processed fats and sweetened foods and beverages, and decreased the amount of healthy fats and proteins in our diet. While preoccupied with fats, we became hooked on sugar. Skip the soda! The average soda contains about ten teaspoons of sugar, often in the form of high fructose corn syrup, which the body turns into glucose and stores as fat. Increases in sugar consumption in the U.S. are off the chart and are contributing to skyrocketing rates of obesity, diabetes, and other health problems.

It took years of trial and error--including an eating disorder--for me to transition from the "all-American" diet, to a vegetarian one, to raw food, and finally to a healthful, varied, and satisfying whole food approach to eating. To overcome my food issues, I finally learned to trust my body, throw out all the rules, and eat what attracted me.

At first, we may be so out of touch and balance that healthful eating seems daunting or even impossible. Go slowly, lovingly, and patiently. As we add more whole, nutritious foods, we will crave unhealthy, sugary, refined foods less, so it becomes easy and natural to eat well. It *is* natural! Through paying attention and self-education, we learn to trust ourselves and become less susceptible to the food "experts," advertisers, and often-misleading books and programs. Trust yourself, and become your own food guru.

Our relationship with food leads us to the deeper issue of our connection with the Earth itself and all its life forms. We would be wise to question where our food comes from, how it is grown, how the animals are treated, and how much fossil fuel and other energy it took to grow, process, and transport. Even within the organic food world there is a huge range, from enormous industrial organic factory farms (as oxymoronic as it sounds) to small, sustainable, living farms. This topic is beyond the scope of this book, but it is one that touches the very roots of our existence. Exploring our relationship with food can help us reclaim our personal and environmental wholeness and integrity.

⊚ Practice Points: 10 Tips for Healthy Eating

1. Breathe calmly and consciously while you eat.
2. Love and Support yourself and your body: Make changes slowly.
3. Pay Attention. How does this food make you feel?
4. Add whole foods: ideally organic, locally grown foods. Focus on healthy, positive additions and changes rather than deprivation.
5. Reduce refined, processed fake-foods, and foods with excessive additives or sweeteners.
6. Choose life. Let your food choices be life enhancing, not a tranquilizer.
7. Protein breakfast. Try eating a healthy, high-protein breakfast for three mornings, and see how your energy feels throughout the day.

8. Rotation diet: Try varying the foods you eat, to help recognize and eliminate potential allergies. (You may need some professional help with allergies.)

9. Educate yourself. Where does your food come from? How is it grown? To reconnect with the land, try growing some of your own food, or join a local food co-op or gardening community.

10. Relax. Don't worry excessively about what you eat, as guilty thoughts can be more toxic than any food. Be patient, compassionate, conscious, and concerned, but not paranoid and perfectionist.

⊗ Contemplation: Making Peace with Food

• Reflect on the foods you eat and have access to. Ponder where your food comes from, who grows it, all the hands who get it to you. Feel gratitude for this gift of food.

• Commit to learning. Put out an intention that you be guided to healthy eating.

BE AN ANIMAL

The bullfrog knows more about rain than the almanac.
- African-American proverb

In yoga, there are cats, dogs, lions, camels, cobras, frogs, pigeons, eagles, cranes, crows, and even bugs. Why are so many yoga poses named after animals? Perhaps it is because animals know instinctively how to move, how to take care of their bodies, and what to eat, and perhaps we can learn from them.

The first time I met Mick, he was easy to spot: full-flowing, graying beard, hand-carved walking staff, rock body, clear eyes, and of course, bare feet. Mick (he would not mind me saying this) is an animal, and I mean this as a sincere compliment. Mick runs a group (he calls it a tribe) called "Going on Foot," which involves taking people back into the forest to go barefoot and "learn how to live again," studying with the guide he calls "Master OGee," or Old Growth. He told me, "The old growth knows how to grow things, so

51

I go there to grow, heal, and learn." Mick had gone to doctors and healers for years, but none could help him with a long list of physical and emotional ailments. It was only after years of learning from the animals, walking barefoot with elk, climbing trees, swimming in icy rivers, and living off the land that he came back into balance.

Life is not really all that complicated, and animals can remind us to stretch, rest, and sleep. Eat (real foods) when hungry, stop when full, keep a clean nest, build a community of fellow Earth critters, make love, and play! Samuel Butler said, "All of the animals except man know that the principal business of life is to enjoy it."[1]

To me, there is nothing more fun than jumping into a clear mountain lake at the end of a hot, summer trek. I once joined a group of hikers who were being led by a member of a local outdoors club. When we got to our destination and I prepared to take a plunge, the leader denied me, saying, "The last thing we want to do is splash around like a little kid and despoil this pristine lake." I grudgingly honored his request but had to laugh when we later saw a deer enter the lake, bounding and splashing along the shore, obviously enjoying itself "like a little kid" (or animal).

I once heard a teacher say that we need to have "dog awareness." Although dogs may take the same walk every day, they have fresh eyes and appreciation, alive to the moment as they smell each and every object.

There are plenty of studies that demonstrate what most of us just know: animals, of course, do have emotions. There are a growing number of reports about depressed elephants, mice showing empathy, and cows holding grudges. Perhaps they are feeling the stress we are causing on the Earth, with human population pressures, pollution, vanishing rangeland, and other challenges.

Still, animals are often more in tune with Earth rhythms and their own natures, while humans are more likely to be overweight, depressed, addicted, or simply disconnected. There are numerous reports of animals saving humans, or responding to tsunamis, earthquakes, and other natural disasters before humans had any idea of what would happen.

My cat Mo is a great teacher--my guru! He is always present, very perceptive and sensitive to energies, forgives easily, and expresses his needs and emotions naturally and unashamedly. He knows how to say no and set clear boundaries. My neighbor had three aggressive dogs, one of which was a pit bull with an ear-splitting yelp. I came to dread gardening, or simply walking across my back yard, with this snarling pit bull charging the short, rickety, insufficient fence. For months, I tried my best to be calm about it, but in truth, my energy field was getting battered and bruised by the violent intrusions and barking blasts. Energetically, I began to feel like a pincushion that had taken too many pins.

Then Master Mo the cat showed up. One day, the neighbor's pit bull came charging the fence with its invasive bark. Without hesitation, Mo drew his ears back, hissed and lunged at the fence, slashing his claws through the spaces in the fence at the startled, rapidly retreating dog. In three seconds, it was all over. Mo had cleared his space, set a boundary, and calmly went on his way.

We humans have strong neo-cortexes and tend to override the reptilian brain and its primitive but effective instincts. We ignore the signals (Enough! No! Run!), often at a price. When we are unable to honor the fight or flight response, we freeze and contract the energy, lock it in the body. We cling to old wounds and trauma, rather than follow the body's natural need to express our feelings or shake it off. This can lead to stress and anxiety at the least, and eventually disease and even premature death in the worst of cases.

We need not idealize animals–they just are what they are and do what they do. They sometimes kill and devour each other, and such is the mystery of life, death, and nature. While not replicating everything they do, they can definitely teach humans a few things about paying attention to our environment and ourselves. We can practice trusting our instincts and intuition, and honoring our deepest needs. The results will make us purrrrrrrrrr.

ꙮ Practice Points

- Practice animal attention, instinct, and intuition. Pay attention to body needs, in contrast to unconscious patterns.
- If you are not comfortable around someone, or do not trust them, do what you need to do to take care of yourself (but

avoid scratching their eyes out!).

- Right now, take a moment and move your body the way your inner animal might move.

∾ Contemplation: Humming Bee Breath

- Humming Bee Breath: (mouth is closed entire time.) Breathe in long and deep through the nostrils. On the exhalation, make a long, soothing, healing, humming sound from the back of the throat, hhhmmmmmmmmmmmmm . . . Do this for 2-3 minutes.
- Reflect: What are two of your favorite or totem animals? What draws you to them, and what are they teaching you?

BE A CHILD

Truly, I say to you, unless you turn and become like children, you will never enter the kingdom of heaven.
- Jesus, in Matthew 18:3

Have you ever watched a baby or young child breathe, or laugh, or cry? They use their entire body, expanding and expressing fully and naturally. They hold nothing back from the present moment of life.

How many of us have been told, "You're being childish!", or "Grow up, would you!"? Well, is this really such a good idea? How about, "Stop acting like an adult!" Many of us adults could benefit by being a bit more childlike.

Children are ancient souls in new bodies. They need guidance, of course, but it is good to remember how wise they already are. They see that we have created a bit of a mess. They see our general unhappiness. They know when we hate our jobs. They watch us eat poorly, mistreat the environment, or go to war. Then we tell them to grow up, listen to your elders, and do as we say. On some level they must know that our world needs them to do something very different. This can create such a painful split in their psyche.

Children are very perceptive and sensitive to their environment, especially while in the womb and during the first few years of life. They are constantly absorbing or downloading stimuli, and this is a natural and healthy part of learning to survive on Earth. Too often, though, we suffocate the life out of them with our own pain, delusions, needs, and expectations. Their young, developing energy fields lack sufficient defenses to filter out these often-toxic energies and programming. It is up to us to take responsibility for what we share.

Rather than rush children along, which often simply inhibits their healthy growth, we can trust their unique process. We can create as nurturing an environment as possible, while assuring their true needs: positive feedback, nutritious foods, and a peaceful home and school setting. Furthermore, what adults really need is to show up for our own lives, take responsibility for our thoughts, actions, and decisions. What children need are parents and role models who are living mindfully, taking care of *themselves*, eating right, sharing their inner gifts, and living authentic lives.

Children can be great teachers when we are astute and humble enough to learn from them. When is the last time you laid on your back and stared at the stars? Or got down on the ground and observed the activities of a bug? An encounter with a frog can make your day! Maybe we should call them *childzen*, for they are the masters of being present. Children are naturally curious, open, intuitive, and loving, and these are the very qualities that many of us need to reapply to our own lives. Children only lose these qualities when they have been around a few years and begin to adjust and surrender to the "normalcy" they experience around them.

While visiting a food bank, a local girl named Ellexa Thengel-Heyman learned that one dollar could buy six meals, and that half the people who visited the food bank were children. Instead of presents for her ninth birthday, she asked for contributions, and later somehow managed to deliver a $20,000 check to the food bank on her birthday. Asked why she decided to ask for donations instead of presents, she answered simply, "Because people are hungry."[1] Amma (Indian woman known as the "Hugging Saint") says, "Once you have attained the state of egolessness, you start seeing everything with the wonder and innocence of a child."[2]

Children can also teach us about emotional honesty, because they feel fully in the moment. They experience their emotions, express them, and then move on. Like animals, they are less likely to hold grudges. And they have so much joy! Madan Kataria, who started the Laughter Clubs of India, writes in his book *Laugh for No Reason* that children can laugh 300 to 400 times a day, while adults are down to about 15 times a day.[3]

As Jack Kornfield says, "Like an innocent child, we can rejoice in life itself, in being alive."[4] We can let children remind us of the innocence, playfulness, and joy of the present moment we used to feel. We can reclaim the magic and mystery of this incredible Earthly adventure.

෨ Practice Points

- When involved in serious duties, situations, or conversations that do not feel life affirming, try allowing your spontaneity, your silliness, your natural tendency to have fun.
- Trust your inner child. Do something just because you feel drawn to it.

෨ Contemplation: Compassion for Inner Child

- Recall moments when you felt vibrantly alive, playful, and curious. How can you practice reclaiming that presence, spontaneity, joy, and play?
- Breathe deeply, and address your inner child. Ask what he/she feels and needs right now. Listen--truly listen--with compassion. Stay in touch.

CREATE COMMUNITY

Where two or three are gathered in my name, there I am in the midst of them.
- Jesus, in Matthew 18:20

The Beatles are the best selling and most popular band of all time. Individually, the Beatles were very good musicians, but together they rocked the world.

The Buddha considered *sangha*, or sacred community, the

foundation for the path to awakening. Something miraculous occurs when people come together with open hearts and minds. We benefit greatly from choosing the company of those who are also seeking truth.

Our predicament is such that we are often lost in loneliness, yet terrified of relationship and community. Certainly we have all been hurt, and relationships always hold the risk of abuse, mutual deception, and greater harm. It's true that the healing path is at times a very lonely one, and so it must be. We each have to face our own inner dramas and demons, and the "dark night of the soul" must be managed internally. Shadows disappear only in the light of presence, and we each have our unique lessons to learn.

While we must do the inner work by ourselves, however, *we cannot do it alone*. Indeed, we are never alone, for we are all interconnected as one great sea. Learning to flow with the other waves is one of our human gifts, and challenges. We can learn to reach out for help, a hug, a compassionate ear, or a word of wisdom. Of course, "connecting" does not mean maintaining an abusive, enabling, or co-dependent relationship. Trusting ourselves, sometimes we do have to say goodbye and let certain people go from our lives. Far more often, however, we benefit by moving towards one another and connecting. You do not find your true and authentic *self* until you connect deeply with *others*.

One morning, a regular yoga student named Sarah--who was going through a divorce--showed up at class feeling quite out of sorts. She remarked, "I slept terribly, and thought about skipping class, but felt it might help." After class, she smiled warmly and said, "I feel so good. And you know why? It's the community." What a profound statement. She didn't credit the poses or the deep breathing--she realized that the group energy made the difference.

Support groups can be very powerful in this regard. Wise and sensitive facilitators can help break open the walls of division and loneliness in one's life. When I found the courage to attend an eating disorder support group, I was stunned and moved by the amount of healing that occurred. I will never forget the liberating feeling of *I'm not alone*, the welcome realization that others around me feel similar pain, confusion, and terror. If you ever feel stuck or half-alive, I strongly recommend support groups for healing assistance.

On a visit to Seattle in April of 2008, the Dalai Lama was asked how America could move away from domination and force, and towards peace and nonviolence. After pondering, he said, "Perhaps the nations' leaders should get together with all their families for a holiday, no agenda or work, just get to know one another. And then later we can deal with the serious things."[1] We can all take an interest in our neighbors and community. Dale Carnegie said, "You make more friends in two months by becoming interested in other people than you can in two years by trying to get other people interested in you."[2]

Gathering places are key in facilitating this need to connect. In many cultures, it might be the local well or watering hole. Here in Washington State, we still have a natural spring just north of Seattle where I like to collect my drinking water as much for the connection with the people as for the pure water itself. In the West, more often it is the church, coffee shop, or bar where we may find each other. There are ever more ways to connect: community centers, men's and women's groups, and even conversation cafes, where a topic is chosen and a safe environment is created where all can speak and listen.

I have heard that reading is not a common pastime for some cultures because it is a solo, isolating activity. People may prefer to gather together in community and celebrate the spoken word through poetry, story, and song. We also have peace potlucks at our home, where people are invited to share food and inspire each other with storytelling, ritual, or prayer. Our house also has a poetry box out front, where we display inspiring poems or quotes for passersby to read. Rather than castles with walls, "energetic moats," and alligators guarding our fortresses, we can create welcoming homes.

We must also bring the me into the we. Too many of us surrender our sense of self when we come into contact with others, or when we enter into relationship. Rather than creating a soup, we can create a salad, each maintaining his or her sense of individuality (our tomato-ness or carrot-ness). We thrive on connection, but it must be a healthy association. Two halves make something less than whole, while two wholes create something even greater.

Intimate relationships greatly raise the potential for growth and healing. What a profound gift to have a committed companion, mirror, and lover to take us places too tender or terrifying to go alone. It's not how well a couple gets along, but how well they don't get along that truly matters. Of course, you won't consciously look for a mate who constantly triggers you and highlights what needs to heal, but how you handle what is fired up in the inevitable disagreements and emotional turmoil is key to transformation.

Connection takes courage. The temptation to turn on the TV and hole up alone is alluring and holds a certain, if illusionary sense of security. Yet it is the safety of isolation, and it carries a price.

We can expand our idea of community to include all of the Earth's creatures. The Lakota have an expression *mitakuye oyasin*, which translates to "all my relations," which are not limited to human beings. The stone, the moon, the cedar, the owl--all are strands in the web of life. We need each other.

Reach out, reconnect, and build sacred community. The world you encounter, while imperfect, may be more kind and loving than you ever believed, and your presence makes it even better.

ᎨᏲ Practice Points

- How might you be the type of friend you wish to attract into your life?
- Practice true, nonjudgmental listening, taking a genuine interest in the lives of others.
- Consider starting a support group, or taking turns hosting community gatherings.

ᎨᏲ Contemplation: Creating Community

- Take a deep breath. What feelings arise with the mention of community? In the past, did community or relationships bring comfort, pain--or both?
- Are your present relationships satisfying, rewarding?

- Visualize the type of healthy, supportive relationships and community you would like to attract into your life. Hold that image and intention.

FEELING FEELINGS

Every morning a new arrival. A joy, a depression, a meanness . . . Welcome and entertain them all!
 - Rumi

Emotions are mysterious and often misunderstood, yet fascinating and dynamic dimensions of our human adventure. Regaining trust in our own emotions and learning to express ourselves in healthy ways is a crucial aspect of self-awakening. We cannot heal what we are unwilling to feel.

Two key concepts here are *connection* and *integration*. When we disconnect or exclude, we often create dis-ease. When we connect and integrate, we heal. Rather than *feel* the feelings we often *seal* them up. As our compassionate awareness encompasses areas of our lives that we previously denied or disconnected from, we become whole.

With yoga, for example, there is the goal of yoking (connecting) body, mind, emotions, and spirit. Yoga invites us to tune in and honor every aspect of ourselves, and as we bring our conscious awareness and essential energy to the body and emotions, we eventually feel better. Feeling brings healing.

It could be said that there are five base emotions, from which an almost-rhyme can be made: mad, glad, sad, bad, and scared—or anger, happiness, grief, guilt, and fear. There are countless off shoots: envy, rage, sulking, joy, loneliness, excitement, terror, and so on.

Every emotion, of course, has its place. Emotions are not the problem; it's the desperate and misguided energies we expend fighting or stifling them. Feelings must be acknowledged, honored, and experienced completely until our very presence transforms and integrates the energies. When you mistrust, fear, and stifle the will and emotions, they may shrivel and constrict--for a while. But life needs expression, and what contracts eventually discharges. Ideally we do not judge ourselves too harshly for some "overly emotional" outburst, when it may only be some long-frozen emotional content finally releasing. Rather than resist and try to re-bury this "lower self" energy, we can appreciate the courageous move towards freedom.

Feeling somewhat ashamed of my sometimes inappropriate behavior during the rebellious years of my twenties, I told one spiritual teacher about "going wild." She gently smiled, and explained that we cannot hold back the feelings and will forever, and that "going wild" was perhaps a necessary step towards healing a rigid and restrained childhood. Practicing kindhearted presence, we can prevent thoughts and judgments from further feeding and conflicting the emotions ("I shouldn't feel this way").

While we sometimes deny our emotions, other times we identify with them. In Spanish it is said *tengo miedo* which literally means "I have fear." In other words, this is temporary; *I have fear*, but *I am not my fear*--the emotions are transitory and changeable. Your own Presence can accompany your emotions, ego, mind, and thoughts. This is the birth of freedom.

It is important to note that there is a delicate but definite distinction between *being with* your emotions and *losing yourself* in your emotions. Yes, take the necessary time to bring compassionate presence to feelings, but if you get lost in the drama, to a point of stagnation, ongoing depression, or analysis paralysis, it may be time to add something different to lift the energy: go jogging, sing a song, watch a funny movie, or anything to shift the emotion. You do not have to stay stuck.

When we denigrate or define the emotions as less than spirit, we suffer a disconnect. In my experience, when I sit in meditation and allow and integrate all bodily sensations, I feel separate from nothing, and a sense of peace and wholeness follows. Sometimes the body simply wants us to show up and take care of it, hear its angst, and have compassion, not unlike a scared child who wants the parent's presence and comfort when it falls. We invite back all the lost "parts" of ourself. Chip Hartranft, in his book *The Yoga Sutras of Patanjali* says, "The yogas of both Patanjali and Siddhartha Gautama regard bodily sensations as a foundation of mindfulness and therefore a direct path to understanding the nature of consciousness."[1]

Men and women may have different innate as well as culturally affected abilities with regards to emotional expression. Boys and girls may have received different messages or permission to access or express their feelings. Yet most of us--men and women--are challenged at emotional literacy.

Our parents, role models, and teachers may not have been comfortable with their own emotions and feelings. They may have allowed us as much emotional freedom as they themselves were able to handle. It's very much like therapists who will only lead a client as far as they are able to go into their own wounds. What was modeled to you? What were you taught about emotions when you were growing up? Did your parents share their feelings openly, unashamedly–which is very different from acting out, venting or abusing? Or, were your parents always miraculously "fine?"

Were your expressions and feelings welcomed? Was crying okay? Sadness? Fear? Anger? Was it even permissible to express those emotions we consider *good*: happiness, joy, laughter? We often inhabit a zone of familiarity--sometimes called a comfort zone, but really *un*comfortable, just familiar--where we allow a narrow range of feelings. Anything outside of that zone jars our energy system. Thus, unrestrained joy or laughter can be disruptive to a depressed energy system, while the same person may dread feelings of anger or grief. We are stuck in half-aliveness, ignoring not only our pain but also our passion, at such a cost!

Emotions become toxic only when denied or conversely, pushed out at others. One of my college students wrote: "I don't focus my attention on the energy within myself. I've learned that I bury my emotions and I don't even realize it until I snap." Like a volcano, we may need to blow a bit of steam to get the lava flowing. Energy expert Barbara Ann Brenna said, "We stop our feelings by blocking our energy flow. This creates stagnated pools of energy in our systems which when held there long enough lead to disease in the physical body."[2]

Deeper, buried wounds and emotions are like prairie dogs, which arise from their holes when it is safe. Recall the beautiful scene from the *Horse Whisperer,* when Robert Redford waits in the field patiently and compassionately until the emotionally and physically damaged horse slowly regains trust, and comes to him. As we provide presence--a welcoming, nonjudgmental, and nurturing environment--what needs to be felt will come out of hiding and present itself. The body, in its wisdom, will show us exactly which layer of energy or emotion it is ready to deal with. We can learn to relinquish our control, time-table, and agenda, and trust the process. We can be *Body* Whisperers, or more accurately, Body *Listeners*.

Feeling and dealing with emotions is one of our greatest human challenges. For thousands of years people have misunderstood that the way to functional living is to *fully express both our pain and our passion.* Even many spiritual teachers suggest rising above our feelings due to their own inability or misunderstanding. This is courageous work, and many of us try to avoid feeling our feelings at any cost. Yet it is *through* our feelings, not *around* them that we integrate, awaken, and live more fully.

ᕮ᠔ Practice Points:

- Whenever intense feelings arise, take a deep breath to invite presence, and check in with your body. At any stressful moment during your day, consider making SPACE for the reflection below.

ᕮ᠔ Contemplation: S.P.A.C.E.: Sacred, Presence, Acceptance, Compassion, and Expression

1. Sacred: Take a sacred pause to give space to whatever feeling or sensation is present or arising.
2. Presence: Ground, and take a deep breath to invite presence. Notice what you are feeling in the body.
3. Acceptance: Allow and feel without judgment. Acknowledge and say hello to whatever you encounter.
4. Compassion: Have compassion for yourself, your body, and the feeling. Listen deeply, with an open heart.
5. Expression: Is there anything you need to do to safely express this feeling or emotion? Or maybe just be present and breathe.

ALLOWING ANGER

I was angry with my friend, I told my wrath, my wrath did end.
I was angry with my foe, I told it not, my wrath did grow.
- William Blake

One of the most challenging emotions is anger. Being human, we all have some of it, buried or otherwise. When you live in a family, culture, or world that insists that anger is bad, you learn to judge or repress it. Thus, many of us eventually deal with our anger by turning it inwards (imploding) or raging and venting it out at the world (exploding.) Neither is optimal or healthy. Imploding anger causes internal disease, while exploding can hurt others or land us in jail! In addition, some of us combine the holding and venting: containing it until it "leaks" out and punishes others in passive-aggressive ways.

My inner work began as sort of an unplanned damage control to what felt like a rupture in my anger storage tank. I was terrified at the rage and countless other feelings that began bubbling to the surface at around age forty. I had no idea what was going on, and just wanted to get on with life and stop *feeling* so much! Dealing with what was bursting into awareness, however, *was* my present life. These feelings had been buried for so many years and they--or unconsciously *I*--insisted that now was the time to deal with them. Sometimes, the only thing I could do was drive around with the windows rolled up tight and scream at the top of my lungs. One day I noticed a pedestrian looking at me with a stunned expression, and realized I had screamed with the window still down! Yet no one was more terrified than I at what was coming up from within.

I had to learn about anger, and to find safe and healthy ways to feel and emote. At a local healing center, the teachers explained that we often feel ashamed and afraid of our own anger, terrified at getting in trouble if anyone knew how pissed off we were. Sure enough, I would smile when I was actually furious. The teachers would constantly remind me, "Run your anger." That made me even angrier, because I had no idea how to do that! After much practice and experimentation, I learned that "running" or allowing anger is less intellectual or even physical, and more intentional or energetic. The teachers taught us to choose a color--red was suggested to represent anger--and visualize it flowing, like hot lava or a clear liquid, throughout every cell of the body, cleansing the energy space and freeing and dissipating the stored fury, as well as the fear and unmet needs that are often beneath it.

Once again, the key is to stay present and feel the feelings. Doing this inner work can be challenging, even overwhelming, and you may need professional assistance. A combination of things may help move anger, including exercise, meditation, counseling, and support groups. It is not an overnight fix, as our terror and rage weave together like energetic scar tissue, or matted dog hair. Compassionate presence is key.

Whether the arising feeling is old anger, fear, shame, or any other emotion, it can be very powerful to be with it in the moment of greatest intensity. Of course, this is when it is most difficult to stay present. But during the height of the spark, there is opportunity for deep feeling, understanding, and healing. You may get a sense of other emotions within it, or an insight into the root of the wounding.

As we cleanse the old layers of resentment, we are more able to deal with present time anger when it arises. In other words, rather than each incident triggering a body full of old unconscious rage or fear, we are able to recognize and trust that whatever emotion that arises is relevant to the moment, rather than decades (or lifetimes) old. Present time anger tends to be more manageable and pertinent. It may tell us: *This salary offer is an insult*, or *Don't let them treat me like that!* If anger is not accompanied by excessive guilt or shame *(I shouldn't be angry*, or *I'm bad for having anger)* it can be used in powerful ways, to say no, set boundaries, or express power. It has some life to it, and can be healing and even motivating when you allow it and let it flow. This is learning to trust your feelings and yourself.

As natural as anger is, we do not want to live there. As the Buddha said, we are not punished *for* our anger; we are punished *by* our anger. Anger and fury grow more toxic the longer we hold on to them. Repressed anger can turn into rage and hate, and this can devolve into disease such as hypertension and heart attacks.

May we not wait to heal our deepest emotional wounds. We can learn to express, purify, transform, and integrate the anger. With presence, patience, and persistence, we can peel back the layers one by one and transmute the rage, until all that remains is our most essential Self.

෨ Practice Points

*   Try to notice whenever anger arises. Take a breath of compassion, and try to stay present.

෨ Contemplation: Allowing Anger

*   Breathe into the body, ground, and ask if any anger would like to show itself.
*   If so, feel it, get to know it. Does it have a color, shape, texture, location in the body? Does it want to say anything, or express itself? Does it need anything from you?
*   Is there any fear, shame, or pain beneath this anger? Welcome this as well.
*   Just be with it, breathing deeply, with compassion. Let it flow like clear, cleansing lava, purifying the energy system.

FEAR NOT

Do not let your heart be troubled, and do not be afraid.
  - Jesus, in John 14:27

Fear is often at the root of anger and many of the other self-defeating emotions. Of all the emotions, fear can be the most, well, scary! It is primal; it links to our very survival and so everyone has to deal with it. Even Jesus reportedly experienced fear and doubt in the moments before his crucifixion.

Among countless fears, some of the most common are: death, public speaking, failure (or success), loneliness, rejection, sickness, conflict, terrorism, and phobias around things like heights, spiders, snakes, and so on.

The United States is not alone in its fear, or course, but it is ironic that the inhabitants of such a rich and powerful country often seem more afraid than many other peoples. We are obsessed with security, with millions of Americans now living in gated communities. Car alarms and home security systems have become the norm. We have insurance for everything, including life itself, yet we are afraid to live. Those who have the biggest walls and weapons are often the most frightened. Perhaps it is because we have more material wealth than many other nations, and we are afraid of losing what we have.

In the deepest truth, there is nothing to fear. Helen Keller once said, "Security is mostly a superstition, it does not exist in nature, nor do the children of men as a whole experience it. Avoiding danger is no safer in the long run than outright exposure. Life is either a daring adventure or nothing at all!"[1]

Yet fear is part of our human experience. American artist Georgia O'Keefe put it like this, "I've been absolutely terrified every moment of my life, and I've never let it keep me from doing a single thing I wanted to do."[2] Still, we do not want to blindly push through the fear or step around it. Our culture equates courage with ignoring or denying fear, but what is needed is a new paradigm, the hero who quietly goes within and faces his greatest terror.

In truth, it is not the outside terror that really scares us; it is what our body holds *inside*. We are terrified of feeling and triggering an emotional explosion. Denied fear forms an obstacle, an energy that exhausts and depletes us and prevents us from allowing grounding, goodness, and grace into our lives. Although it can feel suffocating, frozen fear can be melted and transformed into a gold mine of love.

Like anger, fear can be a natural and present time perception and living message, telling us that something needs immediate attention. A certain amount of cautious concern is even desirable, as in honoring an intuitive hunch that danger lurks, or noticing if we feel unsafe around someone. We may get a horrifying sense that the way we are living is unsustainable. In a human sense, we have every reason to be afraid, and our fear may be worth listening to. We are polluting our air, fouling our waters, warming the Earth, and destroying our nest. We have constructed a world on a foundation of separation and self-indulgence, causing tremendous anxiety. In this sense, our feelings are life gauges on our human dashboard, telling us that something is out of whack, and needs adjusting.

While writing this very chapter, I got a call from a friend back East who was having a panic attack. "I feel so afraid, like I'm going crazy, living on an insane planet, everyone trying to out-do their neighbors. This latest war, the homeless people, climate changes. I feel anxious, tight, sick to my stomach. It feels like we are destroying the Earth, and I don't know what to do about it . . ." Although she felt awful, I honored her for feeling her feelings fully, expressing them, and asking for help. I also wondered how many of us secretly harbor similar fears.

Our bodies are magnificent. We have an efficient sympathetic nervous system for responding to scary and stressful situations, such as an aggressive grizzly bear. We also have a very capable parasympathetic nervous system, which calms us, directing our energy towards digestion and healing. But if modern day living keeps you constantly stressed, as if continually chased by a bear, your body does not get a chance to rest, revive, and restore. You live anxiously and afraid, and age or even die prematurely.

If you are afraid, and have been struggling and relying solely (not soul-ly) on ego and personal willpower to carry the entire load, you have every reason to be afraid. If you can release some of the burden, you can dissolve your ego back into the ocean like sugar into water. When we realize the truth of our Divine and deathless nature, we are liberated from fear and anger and all the emotional angst. Our bodies do die--nobody seems to escape this. Yet we are more than our bodies, and we never truly die. Fear not.

The Buddha reportedly sent his disciples into the cemeteries to sit for some time to learn about impermanence, fear, death, and appreciation of the body and our precious life. Death can be beautiful--just look at the glorious autumn leaves as they depart in a flurry of color, born as tiny buds and dying like proud peacocks. They don't hold desperately to the tree--they let go. Death is the ultimate test in non-attachment. When we become unafraid to face the miracle of death, we are able to make peace with life itself. On the eve of his assassination, Rev. Martin Luther King, Jr., said, "And

I'm happy tonight. I'm not worried about anything. I'm not fearing any man. Mine eyes have seen the glory of the coming of the Lord."[3]

May we honor, learn from, and perhaps even enjoy our emotional roller coaster. It is not a matter of choosing love over fear; rather, it is bringing the fear to our heart. Our essence is love, and fear is simply raw love awaiting transformation. Face your fear; just watch, and then watch who is doing the watching--until the bottom drops out and only love remains.

Practice Points

- Notice moments when your energy contracts or stiffens. How does that feel?
- Is there really present moment danger, or is simply old fear needing attention?
- Try deepening the breath, and grounding your body, and see how that affects your level of angst.

Contemplation

- Ground your body (imagine roots into the Earth).
- Ask yourself: What am I afraid of? Feel your fear.
- Breath of Compassion: Be a loving presence, like an adult holding a child. What does the fear need? Allow it to transform back into love.

PART THREE: BALANCE AND OPEN MINDEDNESS

MAKING PEACE WITH PARADOX

We can open to the world--its ten thousand joys and ten thousand sorrows.
- Jack Kornfield

Which of the following are true?

a. There is only one Truth.	**b. There are many truths.**
a. You know everything.	**b. You don't know anything.**
a. You are perfect as you are.	**b. You are quite imperfect.**
a. Emotional healing hurts.	**b. Healing feels good.**
a. Go within for answers.	**b. Look outside for answers.**
a. Everything is real.	**b. Everything is illusion.**
a. Heaven is here, now.	**b. Life is suffering.**
a. Meditation is effortless.	**b. Meditation is hard work.**
a. You are a Divine Being.	**b. You are body-mind-emotions.**
a. Focus on the joy.	**b. Focus on the pain.**

Paradox is truth within perceived contradiction. Making peace with paradox is a sign of maturity and diminishment of ego, which likes to grab hold of ideas or beliefs, and righteously and tenaciously cling to them as anchors amidst life's storms. The intellect prefers rigid thought forms to uncertainty and mystery.

To keep it simple, let's say that there is an ultimate reality or truth as well as a contextual or earthly reality or truth. Let's touch briefly on each of the questions above, all of which may be true-- unless they are not! First, this very notion of truth:

1. **a. There is only one Truth. b. There are many truths.** Ahhhh grasshopper, of course there is only one truth at the core of all existence, and I will share this in my next, slightly higher priced book. Seriously, while there may be one ultimate Truth, our worldly truth is changeable and depends on circumstances and what feels correct for each of us. Is it "right" to use force or even violence if someone attacks you or your child? Is a lie ever justifiable? One thing is clear: as you lighten your internal load, you find your own truth.

2. **a. You know everything. b. You don't know anything.** As Divine Beings, connected to Source, perhaps we each know, or at least have access to knowing, everything there is to know. In human form, we have limited vision, and that is fine. We simply pay attention to the present moment, trusting that we will know what we need to know, when we need to know it. Not knowing can be opening and powerful.

3. **a. You are perfect as you are. b. You are quite imperfect.** Again, as Divine Beings, we may be faultless. Yet our human selves may experience guilt, denial, hate, fear, grief, ego, and attachments. Such is the perfection of our imperfect human experience.

4. **a. Emotional healing hurts. b. Healing feels good.** Healing can feel both uncomfortable and liberating. As mentioned, we often feel the wounds and swim through their emotional currents as we heal. We may need to agitate the agitation! Yet there is a beautiful and refreshing sensation of lightness that occurs when a shift happens.

5. **a. Go within for answers. b. Look outside for answers.**
Ultimately, you trust the truth of your heart. Yet we all lose
our path at times. When out of sorts, it is often wise to seek the
support of a wise friend, or open an inspirational book.

6. **a. Everything is real. b. Everything is illusion.** Perhaps everything is real, yet every *thing* is illusionary. If there is truly
no separation between you and God, or between anything else
for that matter, how can something be inauthentic? Yet, Earth
is the land of dichotomy and impermanence, where egos reign.
But are human energies such as emotions an illusion? Do they
feel unreal to you?

7. **a. Heaven is here, now. b. Life is suffering.** How often do we
believe things will be better when this or that happens? But,
heaven is here, now, *and* this world can be hellish. Certainly, it
is not easy to overcome suffering and to experience the bliss of
the Divine in human form. Yet when we burst through the veils
of illusion, we can taste the nectar of grace in any moment, in
this very breath.

8. **a. Meditation is effortless. b. Meditation is hard work.** The
heart of meditation is simple: be present, be still, breathe, and
let your attention settle beneath the mind and ego. Yeah, right!
When we become still, all the emotional turmoil we have
saved for another day says, "This is the day!" The mind speeds
up its desperate desire for control, and the body complains and
calls for movement. Yet on some days, there are moments of
effortless bliss.

9. **a. You are a Divine Being b. You are your body-mind-
emotions.** Again, if there is no separation in the deepest sense,
then we are everything, the Divinity and the density. Our right
Mind knows that we are both the Divinity and the humanity.
We are each like individual notes that together make up one
great Song.

10. **a. Focus on the joy. b. Focus on the pain.** Yes, what we
put our attention on tends to grow. But denial, fear, and ego
may invite us to bury that which needs the light of our attention. Wounds and old karmic residue may in fact diminish as

we focus on them with compassionate acceptance. As Yoga comedian Beth Laptides puts it, "When I follow my pain, my bliss follows *me*."[1]

Again, paradox cannot easily be grasped by the intellect, with its limited understanding. When our vision clears, however, we can honor the realm of human perplexity, while moving beyond the small mind's capabilities.

When awake, we need none of the tools presented in this book, which itself is full of paradox. We *are* stillness, breath, and love itself, and presence, power, and passion can emanate from us as naturally as purrs from a kitten lying in the springtime sun.

ᐁ Practice Points

- Notice when you find yourself overly intellectual, defensive, or closed-minded.
- Practice staying open to seeing things from both a human and Divine perspective.

ᐁ Contemplation

- Breathe, rest the mind, and sit in the delight of unknowing. Feel the liberating current of openness.

YIN: PATIENCE AND SURRENDER

The need today is for the awakening of qualities associated with mother-hood--love, compassion, acceptance, and patience.
- Amma

What comes to mind when you hear the word *patience*? Does the concept signify something alien, or perhaps boring? How about the notion of surrender? Does it stir fears and images such as losing, trusting, or giving up control? Or weakness and wimpiness? Does it mean passively allowing anything to happen, even abuse?

We in the West are generally not very accomplished at this patience and passivity thing. We are strongly tilted towards the yang in our culture with expressions like "make it happen," "go for it," and "just do it." Visions of the hard charging CEO, cop, lawyer, or even doctor make for good television, and popular reality shows highlight our competitive culture.

Politicians and pundits take advantage of this fear-based reluctance to yield, with expressions like "these colors don't run," "soft on crime," and "war on terror," and countless offensives such as Operation Desert Storm. Sports teams and mascots include Wolverines, Panthers, and Grizzlies--animals seen as fierce and aggressive. If this yang is not balanced with yin, though, we have, well, what we have--$500 billion war budgets, continuous conflict, and an impatient, pushy, and controlling populace--a terrible price to pay. Controlling everything is exhausting.

I attended an all-boy private high school--a fountain of imbalanced and anxious yang energy. Conversely, I later attended UC Santa Cruz, where our mascot was the banana slug, a beautiful example of yin: steady and slow. The yin-energy is not boring; it utilizes patience and intelligence rather than force, like the blade of grass that threads its way through the tiniest crack in cement. Yin is like the halfback in American football, who yields, weaves, and finds the path of least resistance. Rather than brute force, she knows that success and the length of her career depend on utilizing intuition, ease, and grace whenever possible.

The situation with our returning war veterans (at this moment from Iraq and Afghanistan--our latest tragic wars) is a sad example of excess yang. First of all, war necessitates a heavy yang emphasis--yin qualities of surrender and patience are not encouraged in basic training. When soldiers return from battle, often suffering from depression and Post Traumatic Stress Disorder, it can be extremely challenging to allow the very yin qualities necessary for healing: openness, vulnerability, and letting go--the opposite of what is encouraged on the battlefield. This is especially true since most troops are men, who are given even less permission in our culture to feel, express, and ask for help.

An imbalance is often displayed in hatha yoga, which seeks to harmonize the yin and yang. In the word hatha, *ha* means sun, the fiery yang energy, while *tha* signifies moon, as in be cool and chilling out. If we carry our old yang patterns to the mat, the result is excess push and drive, and insufficient surrender and softness.

Both men and women have masculine (associated with yang) and feminine (associated with yin) energies, and both are necessary in our world. The male psyche and body are built for assertiveness, moving forward, penetrating, while the female psyche and body is better built for receiving, accepting, and nurturing.

Sharon, a massage therapist with nearly 40 years experience, has learned wonderful lessons in patience, paying attention, and surrendering to the wisdom of the body. She says she never forces, "I never push my agenda, but just let the body show me what is next." It is not always beneficial to plan, project, and focus on the future. Like driving on a foggy night, we can trust and allow ourselves to see what is presently in our headlights. Lao Tzu, in the Tao te Ching put it like this, "Do you have the patience to wait till your mud settles and the water is clear? Can you remain unmoving till the right action arises by itself?"[1]

Life seeks balance, and seems to move in cycles. Some say that the matriarchal societies in past eras resulted in an upsurge in patriarchal cultures that are only recently showing signs of receding. Our male dominated world has been suppressing the feminine energies for centuries, with disastrous results, and any time we repress an aspect of ourselves, we all lose. Men and women are suffering from this chest-pounding, heart-attack-inducing lifestyle. Most importantly, we have largely ignored or marginalized the invaluable wisdom of the feminine, which is not weak but strong, and more global and intuitive in its nature and vision.

There is a crucial connection here between the containment of the feminine and the denial of our emotions. Our world has been leading with the head and intellect--more of a masculine trait--and ignoring the intelligence and understanding of the emotions and intuitions--feminine traits. We have feared the feminine, as if it were a threat. It *is* a threat to our unbalanced, overly yang way of life.

When women are empowered and educated, with free choice over their own bodies and access to healthcare and birth control, the need for abortions diminishes, AIDS and poverty rates drop, economies improve, and populations stabilize. Fortunately, things are changing quickly. Some men are crying more, and have you noticed that Spiderman and many other superheroes have a soft side? These are examples of the tremendous transition under way on planet Earth. We are shifting from ego driven doing to enlightened being, from an era of imbalanced male domination to a new age of feminine empowerment.

We can learn from the flowers and fruit, which emerge without force or fight. With patient attention, we can learn to calm our forceful tendencies and surrender to our authentic power and nature's guidance. We can let up, let go, and let God.

ᏋᏇ Practice Points

- Notice when you control or manipulate--how does this feel?
- When it feels like you are pushing too hard, try backing off, trusting, allowing.
- Practice trusting your intuition and feelings.

ᏋᏇ Contemplation: Allowing Breath

- Let the breath go, no control. Just allow and enjoy the free flow of breath. Notice if there is a natural, slight pause at the end of the out breath, before you inhale.
- Reflect: Where in my life do I need to slow down, surrender, and be more patient or receptive in my life?

YANG: ACTION AND ASSERTIVENESS

Do not think I have come to bring peace to the world. I have not come to bring peace, but a sword.
- Jesus, in Matthew 18:15

The yang or masculine energy has an equally important place in the world. We are seeking balance, and there is a time for action and assertiveness, although it works best in tandem with the yin. God cannot ask our boss for a raise--we have to use our voice and speak up.

Yang is like the fullback who, distinct from the fluid half-back, moves forward in a direct line. Even with adversity, he will try to force the ball up field. He generally will not yield, surrender, or pause to reflect. His nature is pushing, not pondering, penetration, not patience. In baseball, it is said, "you can't steal home with your foot on third base."

There is a book called *No More Mr. Nice Guy* by Dr. Robert Glover. For many men--"nice guys" is what Glover calls them--his book is an eye-opener. Glover's argument is that when we "nice guys" (sometimes known as SNAGs--sensitive new age guys) deny our masculine side--often due to shame--we suffer. When we bury our maleness, the life force is also extinguished. As we guys try to be "nice" or unthreatening, we often hold back our natural, authentic, and healthy expression of maleness. In trying so hard to be artificially sweet and gain approval, we lose our own approval. By denying or disallowing the expression of intense emotions such as anger, we end up becoming dysfunctional and passive aggressive.

Many women bravely struggle to get their due respect and place in the world. In some cases women have--sometimes excessively--pumped up their power or push energy. This scares some men, many of whom are already feeling an underlying guilt regarding the suppression of the feminine in which they have participated--consciously or not. Either we men fight back, with ever more masculine force to hold on to our control, or we surrender our maleness. Neither is optimal, as the world needs neither wimps nor warmongers.

Women have also contributed to the male-yang imbalance by excess reliance on male leadership and not taking full responsibility for themselves, often due to guilt, fear, or social conditioning. And many mothers (and men) have in turn raised their children along this paradigm. While men must claim accountability for their insecurity-driven clinging to power, women must take full personal responsibility and leave all victim energies behind.

Kriya yoga is the yoga of action. This is where we stop planning and put into action the idea we have been considering. Yoga poses cannot help unless we actually practice them. The sacred book cannot teach us unless we read it. The benefits of healthy food or breath work are achieved when we actually eat the food and do the breathing. We need the yang, action oriented, take-charge attitude as much as the yin.

We all have yin and yang energies we are trying to balance. Each day brings opportunities to either back off, let go, and surrender, or assert, take charge, and make it happen. The key to a healthy yin or yang is love. Without love, we have selfish and pushy yang and weak and helpless yin.

Being present and connecting with the Self within, we naturally know when doing or being is called for. A healthy use of our masculine or yang energy is a Divine doing to balance the Divine being. While flowing with the stream may get us to the Ocean, swimming upstream also gets us to the Source.

ᘒ Practice Points

The solution for diminished yang, for both men and women, is multifaceted, but might include practicing:
- Knowing there is a time and place to take action.
- Speaking our truth and expressing who we are.
- Go for it. Why not ask for that raise, favor, or date?
- Set healthy boundaries, and learn to say no.
- Be confident, without being arrogant and pushy.
- To heal and balance both the yin and yang energies, try Hatha Yoga, Pranayama, Tai Chi, or Qigong, which help us restore energetic equilibrium to our life.

ᘒ Contemplation

- Alternate nostril breath: This balances the masculine and feminine energies, and is very calming and centering.
- Use the thumb and ring finger of your right hand to take turns blocking each nostril. Start by blocking the right nostril with your right thumb, and breathing in deeply through the left nostril for a 3 to 5 second count. Then, hold both nostrils closed for 1 second, then block the left nostril with your ring finger, and exhale out the right nostril for 3 to 5 seconds. Then again hold both nostrils closed for 1 second, then inhale through the right for 3 to 5 seconds, hold both closed for 1 second, and exhale out the left for 3 to 5 seconds. Continue for 10 rounds. But PLEASE DO NOT STRAIN.

FORGIVE AND LET GO

He who forgives ends the quarrel.
- African proverb

If you have some old wounds, you are not alone. Who among us has not been hurt? Who among us has not held bitterness or resentment? Who has not hurt someone else?

With regards to forgiveness, be forgiving of yourself. Be *for giving* yourself compassion, kindness, and understanding. Can you accept your judgment, sweeten your bitterness, and perhaps even learn to love your hate?

Forgiveness is an invitation to freedom that we can learn to accept. Though uncomfortable, we often stay lost in the emotional quagmire of anger and animosity. My friend Adonnis once told me, "Garbage is supposed to stink. That way we know to let it go." Yet many of us hold tightly, sometimes with an egoist need to be a righteous victim. Since forgiving is a demanding discipline, it must hold priceless lessons, for the intensity of the challenge corresponds with the depth of the lesson and reward.

Personally, for many years, forgiveness did not feel possible. I prayed for release, I wrote letters, and I faced what I perceived as my enemies or perpetrators. I did everything they said in the self-help books, but I still wallowed in bitterness and self-pity. My mother was my biggest challenge; I felt that she had to recognize her faults and express regret. It was always *they* who had to apologize and change. I was the victim.

In truth, it was I who had to take responsibility and release the past. Bitterly blaming others from the past kept me from standing tall and being my authentic self today. What keeps us sick and stuck are not the perpetrators--real or imagined--but our unwillingness or inability to release them and free ourselves.

It is wise, however, to be careful here. Letting go and premature forgiveness can be a form of denial. We cannot get rid of something with which we have unfinished business. We must be clear that we are not running from tender feelings, actions, or lessons. We may wish to give some time and space to the feelings, let them surface into the light, talk to us and teach us. For a while, we may be more angry, more confused, and more pathetic, but an organic process of forgiveness takes time and integration. If we do not turn to face our shadows, they will always be following us.

I clearly and sadly recall the morning of September 11, 2001. The towers had barely collapsed before some people were desperately and angrily calling for revenge and attack. Certainly, there was cause to respond, protect lives, and emote--even vent--our outrage, but calls for introspection, deeper understanding, and eventual forgiveness were often sidelined or even belittled.

If we decide that we create much of our own reality, then we can accept responsibility for ourselves, our lives, and that which happens in our lives. This takes tremendous clarity and courage. When you refuse to forgive, it hurts all of us, but no one more than yourself.

Forgiveness is often *self*-forgiveness, and the release of self-judgment and illusions of both inferiority and superiority. Sometimes you may be the perpetrator, the one who needs to be forgiven by others. In this case, you can decide what brings healing. Do you apologize? Write a letter? Make amends? Or, again, simply forgive yourself?

Auto accidents and other legal issues are wonderful, yet challenging opportunities for releasing blame and victim tendencies. Our egos can get so tightly wound around the "story," and then we have the entire drama of lawyers, insurance companies, and medical providers. If we are not careful, we can completely lose ourselves in the skirmish of right and wrong, cost and compensation. To find sanity, we can somehow stop identifying ourselves as the virtuous victim--or whatever label we cling to--and reconnect with our core.

We do not have to condone what happens in life; we can still request amends, and we can punish or even imprison the biggest offenders. Ideally we arrive at a place of restorative justice, where the needs of both the perceived victim and perceived perpetrator meet eye to eye to express feelings and seek a peaceful resolution. When we see each other and truly know each other, we naturally forgive.

We do not have to wait for others to change (they may be

dead). We can take our power back, perhaps perform a ritual, and decide that we will no longer allow ourselves to be abused by past or present perpetrators. Rubin Hurricane Carter, who was imprisoned--many say wrongly and for racist reasons--for almost twenty years, had to release his hate in order to survive and move on: "If I learned nothing else in life, I've learned that bitterness only consumes the vessel that contains it."[1] When we let ourselves clearly understand the pain and ignorance someone must be experiencing in order to hurt someone else, we forgive. As Jesus said, "Father, forgive them, for they know not what they do."[2]

I recently attended a workshop called The Power of Forgiveness, led by Richard Wiener, a Jewish man who as a child had to abandon his native Germany during the Nazi takeover. Although it took him many years to arrive at forgiveness, he emphasized, ". . . how powerful forgiveness can be, how healing for both the forgiver and forgiven."[3]

Essentially, forgiveness is understanding. Radical forgiveness is seeing and celebrating the perfection in all, and truly trusting the process. Is it possible that there is some order to the universe? Could it be that we come to Earth in part to taste the full range of emotion and experience? Is it possible that we helped create the very events over which we stay victimized? Even if we do not buy into the metaphysical theories, can we be wise and pragmatic enough to realize that forgiveness sets us all free?

⊚ Practice Points: 6 Tips to Facilitate Forgiveness

1. Feel. We may have to wallow in wounds awhile, but pray for a way to bring presence to the pain, and to release the anger. We may need to vent, journal, get therapy, or attend a support group, whatever it takes to move the energy without furthering your or another's wounds.
2. Take Responsibility for your own healing. Decide to not play victim or stay stuck. They don't have to change--you do.
3. Take Action when appropriate: Write a letter (you don't have to send it), or confront the perceived perpetrator. But be careful--make sure you are ready to do this, and have a support person or team. If you do not get the apology you want, you

may in fact deepen the wounding.

4. Learn the Lesson. There is always a gift if we choose to see it. What can I draw from this? Could I have learned this any other way? Count whatever blessings you can. Use this event to become stronger.

5. Clarity. The truth sets us free. Anyone who wounds another is wounded, and is hurting themselves. Can you find empathy for all involved?

6. Patience. There is no deadline; be good to yourself as you go through the process of forgiveness. This is holy work, and like grief, it may take time.

∽ Contemplation: Forgiving Others and Self

- Reflect on someone you feel resentment towards (not yourself).
- Allow and welcome all feelings that arise: rage, anger, etc.
- With presence, empathy, and clarity, look deeply at the person you feel hurt you: what do you see? Take a moment and see this person as an innocent child.
- Do this same exercise with yourself, if there is something for which you have not forgiven yourself. See yourself as a child.
- What if today was your last day on Earth and you wished to clear the slate. Do you need to take any action? What do you need?

ACCEPTANCE AND NON-JUDGMENT

Men are disturbed not by things that happen, but by their opinions of the things that happen.
- Epictetus

Acceptance is a vital component of forgiveness, and an essential mindset for healing and growth. When we can surrender to life and acknowledge that we do not have to control or even understand everything, we can make peace with what is. This is the heart of Zen.

When I was growing up, acceptance seemed like surrendering to the powers that be because they were bigger than I was, and often threatened me with the back of their hand or ruler. I accepted, or really withdrew, but not without heaps of fear, shame, anger, and resistance. This begrudging acceptance lasted only until I was big enough to rebel, resist authority, and eventually claim my own way. But there is a difference between wisely and clearly choosing one's own path and doing so with vision clouded by resentment.

I became further confused when I was working with human rights issues in Central America in my thirties. I became disturbed when I heard about this supposedly evolved idea of acceptance-- did that mean allowing the injustice and poverty in Central America and the rest of the world? Did acceptance mean ignoring the corporations which were pouring toxins into indigenous lands, waters, and communities, or standing by while people were being tortured, raped, and killed? To me, acceptance for the status quo was easy and natural only for those holding the wealth, the power, and the guns.

Terms like acceptance and non-judgment require a spiritual, energetic, and even a pragmatic perspective. They require courage and maturity. We can accept what is, then work to change what we feel drawn to improve with as much passion and efficiency, and as little anger and aversion, as possible.

If we do not recognize something for what it is, we remain confused and judgmental, and judgment is quicksand to any hopes for spiritual growth. What we judge, we are, have been, or will become. Judgment can be a gift, however, as it is simply a trigger that points back to ourselves and what needs healing. If we fail to heed this, we will constantly create or reinforce in our life just that which we judge or do not want. It may not be this minute, or this lifetime, yet universal-karmic law is neutral and consistent.

Who can understand the nature of karma, wounds, and the depths of our underlying spiritual reality? Everyone has their karmic process, and everyone attracts what they put out (although it may not be traceable to anything even in this lifetime). Perhaps life *is* fair, but its very fairness is unrecognizable due to our limited vision. It is important to know that karma is not "bad," and there is another way of seeing karma other than cause and effect, or attracting a "payment" for a past act. Karma is old conditioning which creates a current energy state that attracts an appropriate opportunity to heal and release it, that's all. *The Course in Miracles* says, "All things work together for good. There are no exceptions, except in the ego's judgment."[1]

Judgment is often self-judgment and self-hate projected. It is simply an innocent attempt to feel better about ourselves. Our self-esteem may be so low that our ego needs to see others as inferior. Rivalry and judgment are so ingrained in us that it will take some practice before we can simply see and discern without the destructive blights of separation and superiority. So few of us know the truth and glory of who we really are. As Jack Kornfield says, "Much of spiritual life is self-acceptance, maybe all of it."[2]

Low self-esteem is one of the saddest, most common maladies in our Western world. In my years in Guatemala, I did not see the low self-esteem, ongoing need for approval, and that needy look in people's eye so prevalent in the West. The babies are generally carried on the chest--near the heart--of their Indian mothers. The children seemed to understand that, despite the country's poverty and profound problems, at least they were wanted and loved. When we do not get that early sense of safety, love, and belonging--in the womb and the first year of life--then we experience ongoing angst. Many of us even have judgment day to dread!

Coming to a healthy sense of self-acceptance is a wonderful sign of our spiritual progress. If we can bring compassion to ourselves and every situation, we can say, "Ah, there I go again, judging myself or others. As a protection from pain, I have slipped into inferiority or superiority--how amusing. How wonderful that I am now aware of my judgment." We learn to honor rather than judge the judge.

The master embraces what is. What is the best weather? This weather. What is the best job you have ever had? This one. When the Dalai Lama, who wrote the book, *The Art of Happiness*, was asked to pick the happiest moment of his life, he smiled and replied, "I think now."[3]

⊚⧽ Practice Points

- Whenever you feel some judgment arise, see if you can simply notice it, and gently smile and accept what is.

ᎧᏋ Contemplation: Acceptance

- What are you challenged to accept, right now, just as it is?
- Breathe deeply, and for the moment, just let it be.

NONATTACHMENT AND NONRESISTANCE

There is no goal to be reached. There is nothing to be attained. You are the Self. You exist always.
- Ramana Maharishi

Let's expand on the previous chapter on acceptance. For many of us, the concepts of nonattachment and nonresistance may seem completely alien, as we humans can be possessive and reactive. We are attached to some things but push others away. We want this but not that.

In the yoga tradition, there are five seeds of suffering, known as *kleshas*: ignorance (the main or underlying seed), fear, ego, attachment, and aversion. Certainly all five of these seeds grow intertwining roots. We have already explored two of these: ego and fear, and throughout this book we are exploring the main seed of suffering--misunderstanding or ignorance of our essential Divine nature--which always underlies the other four kleshas. In other words, ignorance feeds ego identification, irrational fear, attachment, and aversion.

Here we explore the last two seeds of suffering: attachment and aversion, which are two sides of the same coin. In Zen, it is said that we must develop a mind that clings to nothing. In many teachings such as the sacred Hindu book, the *Bhagavad Gita*, the idea of renunciation is repeatedly discussed. Our actions and intentions must have no strings attached. We neither push away nor grab tenaciously. We embrace what is. Ideally, we remain so utterly present that nothing can shake our constant, conscious core.

When we do not have that inner anchor, we are vulnerable to other's opinions and our ego's needs. I have heard that what others think of us is none of our business! A therapist friend of mine was delighted one day when a woman called her and said, "I want to make an appointment; I hear such great things about you!" Naturally, my friend brightened to hear this compliment, but then the woman called back a few minutes later to say that she had confused her with someone else!

The Yoga Sutras use the Sanskrit term *vairagya*, (not the male enhancement product!) which relates to neutrality or detachment in all areas of our life. When we do not add reactivity to the *samskara*, or old pattern, we do not extend the cycle of negative karma and suffering. Here, we are unattached to any outcome, including enlightenment. With nonattachment, we can follow the flow, and surrender to the currents and cycles of life itself, the music of our own heart.

With attachment, we pursue, grasp, and cling, from the energy of ego, mind, and fear. What we acquire may bring us momentary pleasure on the physical level, but for every fleeting glimpse of satisfaction, an equal amount of sorrow or suffering inevitably follow. Attachment is like building a sand castle and fighting to keep the incoming tide at bay.

The same holds true for resistance or aversion, the other side of the coin. While we attach to our castle, we curse the waves. When we focus on or push against something we do not want, such as disease, certain people, or depression, we add fuel to the flames. We are essentially inviting it to stick to us, like those Chinese finger puzzles--the harder you pull away, the more you are stuck and the more suffering you create. On hikes, I have noticed that the people who swat the hardest at mosquitoes seem to have the largest following.

Attachments are fed by the ego's insecurities and search for identity, since the ego knows its existence is tenuous and temporary. Many attachments and aversions are also externally influenced by our media and culture, and the chorus of consumerism and competition. We label certain things as more valuable than others, and we have different biases as to "good" and "bad": Muslims (or Christians), people who walk barefoot (or wear high heels), wealthy people (or poor people), small houses (or mansions), or those who are humble and quiet (or assertive and loud).

Everyone wants good health and abundance; few of us want illness and poverty. It is the energy we are talking about here; it is the attachment or resistance to anything that gives rise to anxiety and unhappiness. When we compulsively grab at life, or reactively push something away, we are not recognizing our inherent wholeness. We have lost our center and our Self.

Yet everything holds a gift. What we are compulsively attached to may be showing us our fears, insecurities, or perceived lacks. What we push away may be inviting us to look more closely at what we are resisting. Everything can point us back towards wholeness.

Practice Points

- Notice when attachments and aversions arise.
- Pause and ask yourself: Am I really lacking anything? What am I resisting?

Contemplation: Attachments and Aversions

- What things or people are you presently attached to, or resisting?
- Breathe deeply, and sense your completeness, your power, your love. Then look again at your attachments and aversions.

FAITH AND TRUST

Act as if you are worthy to have what you want, and the universe will prove you correct.
- Alan Cohen

The concepts of faith and trust may seem challenging to many of us, yet they are not so mysterious. What is bizarre is to unquestionably trust societal and cultural norms, or the ego's urgings, and *not* trust our deepest Self and honor our inner cues. We are not necessarily going crazy when we hear inner voices, for these may be the most reasonable and trustworthy guides around.

Here what we are exploring is not blind or overzealous

faith--which can be disguises for escapism, desperation, or attachments--but rather a reasonable trust and a flexible, non-dogmatic, pragmatic faith, based on observation of what works. When we learn to trust our Self, our gut feelings, our passion, and our heart, we open ourselves to miracles. As we practice following the little hunches, we learn that there is such a thing as universal intelligence, and it is us. Then we can loosen the grip and let life flow.

Many of us got the message early on that we are not trustworthy. When our feelings or observations are invalidated, we grow to mistrust ourselves, or others. Children are quite sensitive to external environments. When mother is angry, but she claims she is not, we become confused. If the clergy acts in a less than godly manner, but we are told that they are God's authority figures, we learn once again that we are wrong. All this affects our confidence and self esteem, so we constantly set ourselves up for failure, reinforcing the belief that we are indeed not worthy of trust.

It may take years of practice to begin to understand that our deepest intuition, instincts, and passions are totally trustworthy. It is a learning experience, where we can experiment and observe. When we feel an instinct *(that person does not feel safe)* or a hunch *(I need to read that book or see this movie)*, we can trust it and follow our gut and see how it plays out. Most of us trust our mind and intellect more than the subtle intuitive clues, but our intellect knows only a small part of the situation. Our heart has a more expansive awareness, and the whispering of the soul never lies.

Body wisdom is also trustworthy. I had a yoga student who was obviously in pain throughout a class. When I talked to her about it, she told me she had been thrown from her horse a few weeks ago. Her doctor told her that it was a back strain, and assured her that she could still be active during the healing process, despite the pain. I urged her to trust herself and her own body, and that pain is often simply an indicator that down time is necessary to recuperate, maybe even ponder the significance of the injury. The next week she came back and told me that she had an x-ray taken and found out she actually had a broken vertebra. She had trusted her doctor over her own body, which needed rest and recovery time rather than challenging yoga postures.

There is a reason that the first of the five pillars of Islam is Faith. This faith is an inner knowing that God's face is in everything we see, that the universe is orderly and trustworthy, and that we do not have to manage it! Albert Einstein once said that the most important question we can ask ourselves is this: "Is the universe friendly or not?"[1] The word cosmos means "order," and perhaps universal principles really are predictable, like a good friend you can count on, or at least neutral, as it supports whatever you choose. Select fear, doubt, and failure as your roadmap or expectation, and the universe goes along. Choose joy, success, gratitude, and abundance as your daily thoughts and mindset, and the world again says yes.

Sometimes faith is simply the pragmatic choice between hope and painful defeat. Nelson Mandela said, "Part of being optimistic is keeping one's head pointed toward the sun, one's feet moving forward. There were many dark moments when my faith in humanity was sorely tested, but I would not and could not give myself up to despair. That way lay defeat and death."[2]

Faith requires trust in what the naked eye and the intellect cannot see, trust that there is a purpose to this world, and to our lives, faith that we are part of something bigger than our separate selves, trust that we have created this world not from accident, but with purpose. Trust and faith help us relinquish the fear, open the heart, and return to love.

Another world is not only possible, she is on her way. On a quiet day, if you listen carefully, you can hear her breathing.[3]
- Arundhati Roy

෬ **Practice Points**
- Practice trusting your inner hunches.
- Try surrendering control every now and then. When someone else is driving, for example. try trusting and staying--energetically--on your side of the car!

෬ **Contemplation: Trust**
- Ground the body. Just be. Just breathe. For a moment, release the need to control anything.

- Consider the possibility that the universe is fair and friendly, and that there is nothing you need to do. All is okay, right now.
- Even if you do not believe it, pretend that there is a universal intelligence or God. Express your gratitude, or intention for what you would like to see in your life or in our world. Trust that your prayer has been answered, even before you think or express it.

NEW PERSPECTIVES

Seek the company of those who are still seeking the truth, and run away from those who think they have found it.
- J.T. O'Hara

One of the reasons we put our bodies in odd or extraordinary yoga positions is to see things differently, from a new perspective. This is especially true with inversions, such as headstands, handstands, and other positions where we bring our heart above our head, literally and metaphorically.

You need not stand on your head to gain a new perspective, as there are countless moves and maneuvers one can make to invite a fresh view of reality. You can consciously choose to allow or pursue new ideas or alternative perspectives to greet your eyes, ears, heart, and mind.

Ironically, despite a tremendous, ceaseless, and even excessive availability of information sources, the control of our mainstream media has fallen into fewer and fewer hands. With a handful of mega-corporations grasping the lion's share of the communications industry, we citizens are saturated with a business worldview that inundates us with mantras of the normalcy and necessity of economic growth, development at all costs, and too often, violence and war as a resolution to conflict. We are inundated with the perspectives of the rich and powerful, while the views of those at the bottom of the socioeconomic ladder are underrepresented.

The average American home now has 119 television channels, and each person watches an average of between 3 and 4 hours of TV each day, which often adds more madness to our minds. Studies show that this continued exposure lowers self-esteem, increases depression, and stimulates consumption, materialism, and violence. With tremendous challenges--floods, hurricanes, droughts, food shortages, economic inequalities, nuclear proliferation, and other imperative issues--it is distressing that our news media largely focus on sensationalist, nonessential issues.

Our culture's values often conflict with those real issues of our humanity and our soul, and many of the famous people we admire may not really be all that heroic. Henry David Thoreau said, "If a man walks in the woods for love of them half of each day, he is in danger of being regarded as a loafer. But if he spends his days as a speculator, shearing off those woods and making the Earth bald before her time, he is deemed an industrious and enterprising citizen."[1]

There is good news, however. In the past, one may have needed to wander the Himalayas to find helpful teachings. With the changing Earth energy, spiritual and progressive teachers--many of whom are quite clear and conscious--are appearing everywhere, offering new or ancient knowledge and simple uncommon sense. Thanks to the World Wide Web and instant, inexpensive internet communication all over the globe, we have access to expansive ideas and new perspectives on our environmental challenges, peaceful alternatives to war, and other global healing possibilities.

Much has been said about the escape aspect known as a *geographical*, a psychology term for removing oneself from a place, situation, or relationship only to find that, as Jon Kabbat Zinn says in his book, *Wherever You Go, There You Are*.[2] While it is true that we cannot hide from ourselves, there can be tremendous value in transitions and travels that take us away from familiar places, people, or patterns, and off to newness. This provides opportunities to see ourselves and our world in a different light, from a wider angle. It not only begins the process of self-discovery and understanding others, it can begin dissipating the illusionary distinction between us and "other."

In the support groups I attended while struggling with an eating disorder, the benefits of geographical changes became obvious. Some of the people (most were female) who were bravely and painstakingly struggling to overcome life threatening anorexia or bulimia had found some breathing room, clarity, and improvement by removing themselves from the often dysfunctional or at least triggering situation or space they had been living in. They found a new view.

The limits and even danger of limited perspectives became apparent to me while traveling as a member of several fact-finding delegations to Guatemala, Venezuela and other Latin American countries. We would meet with our Ambassador and other representatives in the U.S. Embassy in each country regarding our policies in the region, but invariably their opinions were as walled off as their fortress. An American we spoke with at the embassy in Venezuela confided that the embassy staff rarely, if ever, left the compound or the elite neighborhood in which it sits. They simply did not connect with the people of the very country in which they were living.

Our entire human experience can be changed with the shift of an intention, attention, or environment. To experience a new perspective, we pay attention, see with new eyes, and listen with new ears. Otherwise, we are staying at an American hotel in Puerto Vallarta eating burgers, rather than meeting native Mexicans, tasting authentic local foods, and listening to traditional Mariachi music. Our worldview remains shallow and insignificant. When it comes to healing, if you feel stuck, or if there is some aspect of yourself that you are interested in changing, try doing something different.

We need not venture off to India, as every moment offers opportunities to see and hear anew. Find the courage and willingness to listen within, hear that present yet primordial perspective, whispering truth and love. It is the voice of wisdom that resides in your own heart, awaiting your re-discovery.

ஒ Practice Points
* Today, see, sense, and listen with an open mind and heart.
* Do something different today--bike, drive, or walk a new route.

ஒ Contemplation: New Perspectives
* Consider a time when you put yourself in a new position, or

place. What did it teach you about yourself and others and life? Honor your courage.

- Where in your life might you benefit from allowing a new perspective?

CHALLENGE YOUR BELIEFS

The Holy Spirit will teach you to perceive beyond your belief, because truth is beyond belief.
   - A Course in Miracles

We continue with this theme of opening to new perspectives, and the liberation this offers. We've already explored the roots of suffering, and how the root of attachment grasps deep into the soil. Well, is there anything we cling to more desperately and defensively than our beliefs?

To what beliefs do you adhere? Are you willing to change your mind, or challenge these beliefs? Would you consider discarding some or all of them if it would bring you freedom?

Beliefs are hard earned, one might argue. It has taken us years, decades, or even lifetimes to learn the treasured lessons, and acquire the knowledge necessary for survival and abundance. We may have invested in costly education, and our beliefs and knowledge offer us competitive advantage.

Many of our beliefs are unconscious. As children, we are naturally programmed for survival, downloading cues from our environment. Yet we also take on many harmful beliefs ("I'm not good enough"). Our evolution depends on our willingness to release the old and bring in the new. Do you hold all the same beliefs you held as a child? Ideally, we have let go of the beliefs we no longer need, such as, "boys don't cry," or "girls don't get angry." If we hold true to rigid and outdated--if they ever had a date--thought forms, we are stuck. People once believed the world was flat. Some of our most cherished minds, such as Albert Einstein, were believed to be slow or stupid.

Of course, religion can be the dominion of fixed beliefs

and closed minds. It can also be the place of openness and expansiveness. We can stay present, trust ourselves, and ask: What serves me? What makes sense today, or in this very moment? Often we are too closed, or too open. We need openness without naiveté. With regard to spirit, for example, if too open and without "filters", we are vulnerable to others' convictions, and could end up involved with a strict religious group or even a cult. We have no sense of our own truth and we grasp whatever presents itself. If too closed, we are stuck on old beliefs, unwilling to even consider that spirit, God, or another reality exists, or that there is another way of seeing or being. Neither extreme is healthy.

Perhaps the ideal would be to move beyond all beliefs, since all thought forms are capable of stagnating and morphing into solidity and self-righteous rigidity. Now, it may seem unrealistic and impossible to imagine life without at least some guiding beliefs. But imagine a truly enlightened being: so utterly present and awake that she knows intuitively how to be, respond, and act in each situation. She needs no history, for she is wholly present. This is the Amma, Jesus, or Buddha, the woman or man so alive and awake that no unyielding thought form could survive in their enlivened presence.

A baby elephant's mind can be trained by tying its leg to a stake, so that even as an enormous adult it will not challenge the belief that it can't tug itself free. The bondage is in its faulty belief, and it does not know its own strength, just as so few of us realize our own limitless power.

William Wordsworth said, "Habit rules the unreflecting herd."[1] Without a pause to breathe and reflect, we fall into the same old patterns. The well-worn path of least resistance is chosen, even if it is someone else's footsteps. Does this mean that the study of history has no place, that we need not look back nor forward, just be here now? Few of us are so clear that we can yet entrust ourselves so confidently to our sense of present Self. Looking at what has happened in the past can reveal cycles, patterns, and invaluable perspectives. Yet we need not limit ourselves by them, for we are making history today, with every thought, word, and action.

There is a Zen saying, "Don't seek the truth. Just cease to cherish opinions." We have Democrats, Republicans, Progressives, and Independents who no longer hear what the other side says, even if at times it makes more sense than their own version. Basically, we are talking about humility, staying open, unattached. Can we easily and naturally let go of yesterday's ideas as we transition to today's changing world?

We buy into the tragic lie that we humans are not caring and compassionate beings. We defiantly defend capitalism, a system which seems to invite or even incite the worst elements of human nature--greed, competition, consumption, and the resulting domination and devastation of the earth. We take for granted that some will be wealthy and some will be poor and struggling. We accept a wealth disparity where the top five percent of Americans owns more wealth than the bottom 95 percent.[2] The taboo topic of redistribution of wealth has been buried or outright attacked and labeled as socialist (even though we may not know what that means). But it is natural and necessary that we question these beliefs, face our fear of change, and learn to share.

Personally, when I feel myself clinging to a belief or opinion and my need to be right, I feel an energetic restriction in my body. My voice changes and my heart hardens. I do not care much for myself when I am being defensive. Yet there is such relief and freedom in saying, *I don't know*, or *perhaps I am wrong*. In fact, I would bet that when I look back at this book in the future, I will see things that I disagree with, as I evolve and as my beliefs and ideas change. Jonathan Swift said, "A man should never be ashamed to admit he is in the wrong, which is but saying in other words that he is wiser today than yesterday."[3]

Attentive listening is key to challenging our beliefs. When we listen, we can be totally present. Listen with your heart, your mind, your whole being, rather than obsess with what you will say next--that which your chattering ego thinks is clearly more important than what you are half-hearing. This is also incredibly satisfying and healing for the one being heard. Talk show host Larry King once said, "I never learned a thing when I was talking."[4] We can listen to our children, our pets, to the trees and rocks and the Earth itself. Teachers are everywhere!

Our world is changing so quickly. Many old beliefs no

longer apply, and a new consciousness is being born. Native peoples, once feared as uncivilized, are now honored for their wisdom. Slaves helped build the "White" House, where a dozen ex-Presidents owned slaves; in 2009, a Black man became the newest resident as our 44th President. For generations, women could not vote, but are slowly claiming their rightful power. Indeed, we are presently sprouting roots of a new paradigm that encourages and supports our deepest nature.

Our survival depends on loosening our grip on frozen beliefs, opening the possibility for genuine democracy and deeper awakening. Without the distortions of our rigid preconceptions, the mind clears, and we are able to reflect the deepest truth.

⊚ Practice Points

- Notice when you feel defensive, argumentative, or self-righteous. How does this feel?
- Try softening, listening, being totally present and open to learning something new.

⊚ Contemplation: Open Mind

- Breathe deeply and reflect: What would it feel like to be completely open and unattached to my beliefs?
- Just sit for a moment, totally open, receptive to learning something new, perhaps right this moment.

MYSTERY AND HUMILITY

Do you think I know what I'm doing? That for one breath or half-breath I belong to myself? As much as a pen knows what it's writing, or the ball can guess where it's going next.
- Rumi

Essentially, what we have been exploring in the last two chapters, "New Perspectives" and "Challenge Your Beliefs," is humility, being open to the mystery. While we can calm the mind and awaken our heart to wholeness and brightness, we are presently in imperfect, sometimes sloppy, human form.

Again, we all want our power and assertiveness, and enough confidence and healthy willpower to take appropriate action in our world. Yet we are wise to balance this healthy sense of self with a non-egoic power, bowing to that which we do not presently understand. At the Seattle Green Festival in 2008, Francis Moore Lappé spoke of "bold humility," honoring all our imperfections, but moving through our fear to power and greatness.

One of the New Age buzz phrases is that we create our entire reality. We are certainly creating with each and every thought, word, and action. Yet perhaps this notion of creating everything appeals to, or stems from, our inner control freak. We like to believe we have complete control, but do we? We have seven billion other human beings on the planet also thinking, creating, and acting, along with billions of other creatures and their creative energies, not to mention the totality of God Himself-Herself interacting as a part of all this! Clearly, we all affect each other in countless ways. If I am the only one visualizing world peace--or world war--the majority may win.

A friend of mine shared a lesson in humility, learned while she was working at a Christian retreat center. Each week one member of the staff took a turn leading a Sunday ritual. There was one very timid member of the staff who hardly ever spoke, and when it came to her turn, people wondered what she might be able to do. When everyone gathered, she looked down and shyly whispered, "Today, we are going to wash each other's feet." And so they did. My friend said it was one of the most profound rituals they had ever experienced. What can be more respectful and connecting than washing each other's feet, as Jesus had done and said, "He who humbles himself will be exalted."[1]

The Qu'ran (Koran) encourages Muslims to dedicate themselves by frequently prostrating, thus relinquishing arrogance, while nourishing humility. Zen teacher Shunryu Suzuki tells a story about an obstinate teacher who worked to overcome his stubbornness by forcing himself to bow over and over to the point that he developed a callus on his forehead![2] Bowing and humility are not about humiliation or self-effacement, which serves nobody. Humility relates to humus, "of the earth." Like a seed that falls humbly to the ground, takes root, and becomes a mighty tree, by bowing we can actually elevate ourselves and each other.

Allow me to share a personally humbling yet liberating experience, about a visit to my family in my birth town of San Francisco in the fall of 2006. I had been doing lots of inner healing work, but each time I visited my family there seemed to be no change or shift in our relationship--same old confusion, triggers, dramas, and conflict. So many times, I considered severing the relationships with my family; I always feared, resisted, and judged *their* energy, *their* control, *their* anger and meanness. So, every time I visited or spoke with them, I carried mountains of anger, apprehension, and resistance.

This time, I had a new strategy. I vowed to keep my heart open, not take anything personally, not fight back or judge. The results were miraculous, and I watched my relationship with my family transform itself instantly. I was no longer foolishly feeding the fire with my nasty fuels of resentment and fear. The great Tibetan sage Milarepa said, "You menace others with your deadly fangs. But in tormenting them, you are torturing yourselves."[3]

I realized, with much humility, that they had often been reacting to *my* judgment, *my* fear, *my* anger, *my* meanness, and *my* smallness. I always had a self-righteous attitude about how they were the problem, not yet evolved like me! In truth, we were all the problem, and I was the part I needed to worry about and heal. As I began sending love rather than fear, they returned it in kind. Previously, I had not given them space for other options, for I was energetically in their space trying to control them!

Total control leaves no space for the mystery of it all. Being human is mysterious, is it not? If we think we have all the answers, we are probably being conned by our intellect. Minds are poor masters, and rare is the master of the mind.

Confusion and bewilderment, like emptiness, can be rich and wonderful places to be or begin from. When we think we know it all, we slam the door in God's face. With humility, we ironically invite Divine guidance and inspiration to lead us further and deeper than our little minds are capable of going. In our heart of hearts, perhaps we are capable of knowing it all.

We can quietly recognize and acknowledge that we are as amazing and unique as everything and everyone else. We can remain humble and open, even as we claim our essential glory, greatness, and Godliness.

ᔆᕀ Practice Points

- Stay open. Practice "bold humility."
- Be aware of times when your vanity jumps into action with feelings of superiority and arrogance.
- Be open to that which you presently do not know.

ᔆᕀ Contemplation: Bold Humility

- Reflect: Does being humble carry with it a certain feeling of vulnerability?
- Is it possible to be strong and humble at the same time?

PART FOUR: ENERGY

GROUNDING

To lose our connection with the body is to become spiritually homeless.
Without an anchor we float aimlessly, battered by the winds and waves of
life. Disconnection from the body is a cultural epidemic.
- Anodea Judith

Grounding is the energetic connection we make with the Earth. For some of us, grounding is easy, not something we are even aware of. It is our natural way of being. We feel reasonably safe and comfortable in the world and in our own skin, and generally feel present to others, our surroundings, and to life. We all know people like this. They seem to trust that they are here for a reason, and know that they have a purpose.

For others, grounding does not come easily. We may feel scattered, unsafe, or insecure. Fear may keep us wary and light on our toes, ready to run and escape from potential threats--real or imagined. We may be hesitant to root too deeply, for fear of being like a tree in timber-cutting country, or a sitting duck.

Body type is sometimes, but not always, a hint to our grounded-ness. Heavier people are often more grounded (sometimes excessively so), while others may be thin, again, as if we do not want to make ourselves too big of a target! Using myself as an example, at 5' 8," I have never weighed more than 135 pounds. I have often resisted being on Earth, sometimes feeling as if a mistake were made, like I was abandoned or dropped off on the wrong planet. Being very sensitive to energy, combined with an uncomfortable and unstable childhood environment, I thrived--or at least survived--on movement, hesitant to plant deep, sustaining roots. For much of my life, I changed locations, jobs, and relationships easily, and had difficulty manifesting any lasting stability in my life.

As with learning about anger, when I first heard about grounding in meditation classes, I had no idea what they were talking about--I literally felt no connection. At the same time, I found myself either *resistant* to--or alternatively sometimes *attracted* to--things that would help ground me: nature, dancing, yoga, tai chi, and even heavier foods or grounded people.

My cat Mo is my grounding and energy teacher and meter. If I have anxious or ungrounded people over to my house, my cat Mo will take off; he's outta there. But he will easily sprawl out on the floor when we have a grounded group of friends over. I sometimes even bring him to my group yoga classes, as he enjoys the peaceful, nourishing, grounded energy.

Why is grounding important? Essentially, for the same reasons being present is important. If you do not come fully into your body, bring your energy downward into the feet and Earth, you do not allow yourself the full human experience. You remain wishy-washy, unable to establish a foundation and allow the grounding energies of the Earth to nourish you. Fear may lead your life. Not grounding *keeps* you feeling disconnected, unsafe and insecure--not a healthy cycle.

Many of us have our energy and attention in the head and mind. We may be spacey, scattered, anxious, or overly busy. For example, a woman may have tremendous ideas and imagination, but if she is ungrounded, she will be unable to bring those ideas into fruition. She will always have that great book residing (and perhaps rusting) in her head. This, my first book, came only after many years of ideas, and then ten more years of healing, yoga, and other grounding work.

To be truly successful, we come fully into the body. All successful and thriving people, whether athletes, politicians, teachers, or actors are generally well-grounded people. They know how to bring that creative energy down from the head, through the heart and connect with the nourishing foundation of the Earth.

⏝ **Practice Points**

• When you find yourself thinking or worrying excessively, bring your attention down into your body, and feel your feet.
• Make time for a short walk--maybe even barefooted!
• Try yoga, Tai chi, Qigong, dancing, hiking, gardening, being in nature, or getting a massage--whatever grounds and nourishes you.

⏝ **Contemplation: Be a Tree**

• Breathe, and imagine yourself growing roots, from the core of your body and from your feet deep down into the Earth, like an old growth tree. Feel the nourishing support of the Mother Earth beneath you.
• Assure yourself that you are safe and secure, here, now, in your body.

CHAKRAS

". . . the activities in the various chakras influence our glandular process, body shape, chronic physical ailments, thoughts, and behavior. By using techniques such as yoga breathing, bioenergetics, physical exercises, meditation, and visualization, we can, in turn, influence our chakras, our health, and our lives."
- Anodea Judith

Chakras are subtle energy centers that extend from within the area of the physical body out into the aura, or energy field. They filter, store, and process energy (prana) and information, and affect the physical, emotional, and energy body. They correspond to the energy channels, called *nadis* (like meridians), especially the main energy channel along the spine, the *sushumna*.

In the West, chakras are coming into mainstream teachings, a gift from the East. Buddhists, Sufis, Hindus, Yogis, and Taoist teachers have all known of chakras for centuries. Chakra is a Sanskrit word meaning wheel or disk, and this is fitting, because like our computer disks, we sometimes benefit from reformatting our software, cleaning out the old, outdated beliefs and patterns.

Chakras will not show up on an x-ray or an MRI, but there are people who are intuitive enough to sense or see the energy and colors with the naked (or inner) eye. Sensitive *Kirlian* photography can help us glimpse photos of our energy field and whatever colors are present in that moment (they change instant to instant). Opinions differ as to how many chakras, or energy vortexes there are in the energy field, but most agree that there are at least seven major chakras. They are aligned from the top of the head, down along the spine to the area near the base of the tailbone, or perineum.

Do we need to know about chakras? Probably not. My cat does not know how many chakras he has. If we simply do what feels good, we will most likely balance the chakras. Awareness of the chakras, though, may help us tune in to the subtle energies, know and understand ourselves better, and facilitate healing on all levels. The energy of the chakras needs to move, or spin actually, to be healthy and effective. Trauma, abuse, emotional turbulence, stagnant (or frenzied) energy, faulty beliefs, and many other factors affect the activity of each chakra, and therefore our health on all levels.

A color is often associated to each chakra, which represents a slightly different energy vibration or frequency. Like the rainbow, the chakras go from red at the first chakra (most dense) to violet at the seventh chakra (least dense, or highest frequency), but again, the colors change. Here is a brief overview of the chakras:

First chakra (earth element), located near the perineum or tailbone, is our root chakra, the connection with Earth, primal urges, and survival of the body. Fear and insecurity are the main blocks to a healthy first chakra. Trust, safety, and grounding (nature, walks, dance, etc.) help heal it. Red is the color associated with this chakra.

Second chakra (water element), a couple of inches below the navel, is the center of emotions, creativity, pleasure, and sexuality. Guilt, shame, and lust may imbalance this one. Allowing play and pleasure in your life, feeling your feelings, body movement, and healthy expressions of your sexuality heal this chakra. Bright orange color.

Third chakra (fire element), at the solar plexus, is the center for personal power, self-confidence, and healthy expression of will and ego. Again, guilt or shame, or overconfidence or arrogance, seem to be the main blocks here. You heal it by taking appropriate action, raising your self-esteem and confidence, and knowing you can handle life, with proper humility. Bright yellow.

Fourth chakra (air element), or heart chakra, at the middle of the chest, is the center of connection, love, gratitude, and compassion. Grief, judgment, fear, and anger close the heart chakra, while loving, giving, and receiving, as well as community and connection heal it. Bright green color.

Fifth chakra (sound element), at the throat, is the center for communication, self-expression, and speaking truth. Gossip, lies, "swallowing your words," and untruth distort this center, while living an authentic life, active listening, singing, toning, and self-expression heal it. Bright blue color.

Sixth chakra (light element), or third eye, at the brow, is the center for intuition, discernment, clear seeing, and healthy mind. Illusion and self-importance are enemies of this chakra. Meditation, visualization, and being willing to see what truly "is" help balance this chakra. Bright indigo.

Seventh chakra (thought element), at the crown of the head, is the Divine connection, and center for faith, inspiration, and guidance. Main blocks are rigid beliefs, or conversely, being too open with inability to filter information, making one vulnerable to another's manipulations. We heal it by releasing stuck beliefs, not attaching to ideas, practicing a pragmatic faith, while following our deepest truth. Bright violet color.

Each chakra has a balance point, as well as both an excessive and deficient challenge. We already mentioned that an ungrounded or deficient first chakra person may live in the head, while one who is excessive in the first chakra may be grounded, but could also be a couch potato. An excessive second chakra could result in exploding emotions, hedonistic activity, or sexual addiction, while one with a deficient second could show inability to feel feelings, move the body, have fun, or allow healthy sexual expression. An excessive third chakra person is controlling or manipulative, like the type A, self-important, hard-charger who is full of yang and fire energy, stopping at nothing. The person deficient in the third chakra lacks confidence and will, may feel helpless, and is easily walked over.

A person with an excessive fourth chakra might be judgmental, jealous, or codependent, while a closed fourth chakra could result in disconnection, loneliness, or despair. The person with an excessive fifth chakra, might be dishonest, untrustworthy, speak too loudly, or dominate the conversation, while the deficient fifth chakra person speaks too softly or does not feel able to express him or herself. Excessive tendencies of the sixth and seventh chakras might be delusional, naïve, or egotistical beliefs, while deficiency reveals a person holding rigid beliefs, lacking faith, and living without purpose or direction.

There are countless ways to heal the chakras. The lower chakras are healed by taking care of the body (perhaps doing yoga, tai chi, or Qigong, or receiving bodywork), expressing emotions healthfully, allowing healthy pleasures, taking appropriate action, and connecting in community. The higher chakras are healed by speaking truth, singing, listening to soothing music, living authentically, meditating, reading sacred texts, and opening to new ideas, among many other possibilities.

This is a very challenging time on Earth for our first chakra, and when our root is damaged, all the chakras are affected. The physical, economic, and environmental changes happening in the world are testing our ability to stay grounded in our bodies. When scared, we tend to pull up roots and head to higher chakras (although we may also lose our Divine connection as well). To help heal this world, each of us must stay present and balanced in our chakra system, connected to our personal body, the planetary body, and our deepest Divinity.

෨ Practice Points

* Try exploring the balance in each chakra between excessive and deficient:

Excessive	Deficient
1st) sluggishness	ungrounded
2nd) emotionally or sexually overreacting	closed down
3rd) self-important	unimportant
4th) smothering	separating
5th) talking too much	shutting-down
6th) delusional	lacking imagination
7th) naïve or gullible	rigid beliefs

෨ Contemplation: Chakra Colors

* *Breathe color into each chakra, cleansing and balancing each energy center:*
* Perineum / Red: Release fear. I am safe. I belong here, now.
* Beneath Navel / Orange: Release guilt. I Feel. I allow movement, pleasure, and healthy sexual expression.
* Solar Plexus / Yellow: Release shame. I allow healthy power. I take action. I have a healthy sense of self.
* Heart / Green: Release fear and grief. I connect. I give love and receive love.
* Throat / Blue: Release lies. I express myself, speak my truth.
* Brow / Indigo: Release illusion. I see clearly, and my mind is calm.
* Crown / Violet: Release confusion and attachments. I allow guidance, and I am open to new information. I trust my Self.

LIFE FORCE ENERGY

A beautiful or peaceful thought, a thought such as love, is the greatest source of human energy.
 - Swami Veda Bharati

Prana and chi are two of the many words used to describe life force energy. These energies help us cleanse our energy systems, and wash the debris from our channels so we can maintain the flow and aliveness in our body.

It is the movement and *quality* of energy, not necessarily the *quantity* of energy that counts. We often say *I need more energy*. In truth, we have everything we need, although the energy may be blocked or stagnant. Furthermore, we often absorb energies around us that diminish, dull, or deplete us.

A friend of mine performed an experiment. She cooked a pot of brown rice, then place an equal amount of rice in two carefully chosen, identical, sterilized glass jars. She placed a label on each jar, facing in towards the rice. One said, "You are beautiful rice. You will have a long life." On the second, she wrote, "You are horrible rice. You will perish quickly." She placed them in light-proof bags in the refrigerator, and after 90 days, she pulled them out. The first one smelled fresh and edible, as if cooked the day before. The second one was green and moldy! Others have done similar experiments with plants and water. Again, it is the quality of energy that counts.

In the simplest of terms, we can learn to seek those energies that feed, nourish, and sustain us, and avoid those energies that harm or drain us. When our consciousness is lower than the surrounding people or energies, we might wish to allow ourselves to be lifted by those energies. For example, if we are strolling through an old growth forest, or amidst a group of enlightened healers, we may want to surrender to the prevailing energies. On the other hand, if we are with lower conscious energies, such as people in fear or self hate, we would be wise to ground, maintain our own space, and not match the denser energy vibration. I already mentioned Mick, who still lives much of his life in the old growth forests of the Olympic Peninsula. He told me that 72 hours is the most he can handle in the cities, where the energies of the "civilized" world dull and drain his life force.

Each of us sees the world through the window of our energy field, or aura. If your life force is stuck, and your energy field is soiled with unresolved trauma and pain, you will see the world in one way. Like looking through a dirty window, regardless of what is really going on outside, you will see muck or negativity. But when the window is clear, when you have cleansed enough of your old pain and delusion, you will see with clear perception. You may still see the world's pain, but you will not be quite so enmeshed with it.

The world's energy, in any event, is simply an extension of each of us. Our world peace activism is best rooted in our spiritual practice. Healing is just this: using the always-available life force energies to strip and purify us to the core of who we are. Again, breath work is one wonderful way to move the life force energy through the system. Conscious breathing connects us with the prana, which we can follow like a river to its Source. Prana--also known as chi--is like a bridge between the physical world of form and the deepest reality of Spirit.

We just mentioned chakras, which are energy centers that receive, assimilate, and express the life force energy. The yoga belief is that when the chakras come into alignment, a specific, transformative type of life force energy called *kundalini* is free to dance its way from the base of the spine up through the chakras, stirring our consciousness to greater levels of wakefulness, joy, and bliss. While beyond the scope of this book, let's just say that that kundalini carries quite an energy jolt to the more dense human energies. It is believed that this "coiled serpent" of energy resides at the base of the spine and may be consciously or spontaneously awakened to travel up the spine and provide us a taste of Divine grace.

Like breath work, running kundalini energy can be somewhat overpowering to the unsuspecting or ungrounded person, so be mindful when using this powerful energy. There are many teachers who guard the secrets of kundalini, or who will not teach them to novices, sometimes with good reason, and sometimes out of fear or even for egotistical reasons. Kundalini energy is not to be feared, as it is natural. But we are wise to respect it and take responsibility for using this subtle yet profound energy, as its frequency is much higher than what most of us are accustomed to. If you are called to try it, please see the following kundalini meditation. Also consider working with a qualified kundalini teacher, and doing the prep work by healing the body and as much of your inner emotional wounds as possible.

Whether it is music, dance, laughter, or meditation, you increase the flow of life force through your body and energy system by doing whatever works for you, anything that stirs feelings of genuine joy, love, and peace.

ගුණ Practice Points

- Notice what kind of situations, activities, people, or surroundings drain or deplete you.
- Notice what kind of situations, activities, people, or surroundings feed and nourish you.

ගුණ Contemplation: Kundalini Energy

Note: Kundalini energy is a powerful, high vibration energy that rises from the base of the spine. Please be very present and grounded when using this energy. Be aware that it may stir up lots of feelings, and "stuff" in the healing process.

- Breathe, and sit comfortably. Relax the body.
- Ground, from center of body (the navel area) down through first chakra (energy center near tailbone), to core of Earth.
- Run Energy / Purrrr: Imagine, and allow prana to run throughout the body, down through crown chakra at top of head, down spine, arms and legs. Also, up through feet and legs, up the spine. Imagine a cleansing, healing flow of energy.
- Kundalini: Allow a light, bright, gold energy to stir and move up from the base of the spine. You may feel a subtle tingle as you allow this energy to flow up along the entire spine. No effort, just ground, be, and allow.
- Breathe: stay present with your body as you run this profound energy (you would not leave your house with a candle lit.) Allow it to transform any physical, emotional, or belief blocks in

your energy system.

- To finish: When through with your meditation, visualize a cool blue light running down from the top of the head, down the spine, cooling or dampening the fire of the kundalini, putting it to sleep at the base of the spine. Feel the peace, love, and joy that you are. Stay grounded as you continue with your day, and notice what might have been stirred in you.

IMAGINE THAT

We are what we think. All that we are arises with our thoughts. With our thoughts, we make our world.
- The Buddha

Imagine your dream job, or if you prefer--no job! Visualize a world without suffering, where no one is destitute or depressed, and everyone experiences joy and abundance. Imagine tremendous and unprecedented shifts in consciousness, and an enlightened and radically responsible global community. Imagine a world where bombs, borders, and barbed wire are replaced with peaceful community. Foresee honoring of the various cultures, religions, and life forms, revisiting traditional wisdom and time-tested connection with the land. Or dream of something totally new, a flourishing of grand ideas. Envision living in balance with the Earth, environmental rejuvenation, waters replenishing, air purifying, forests regenerating, species rebounding.

Imagine a world at peace. Is this an unrealistic dream? Are those who talk of world peace immature and idealistic? Or are they simply refusing to "grow up" and relinquish their childlike and God-given ability to visualize what they want to see? Are they indeed brilliant, knowing that their songs, images, and hope might just help awaken and encourage millions of others to imagine and therefore help create a world without war?

Children do this creative imagining naturally and effectively. The doll or the toy they want often begins as a vision. They will think about it, visualize it (and ask for it). All ideas--positive or negative--begin as an image, a spark, a daydream. As Albert Einstein put it, "Imagination is more important than knowledge."[1]

When I meet people who seem to suffer from low self esteem, their voice and energy tell me that they believe they are unimportant. I have had students or workshop participants whose names I simply could not remember. Certainly, my mediocre memory was a reason, but I also came to see that sometimes the person had the belief, fear, and expectation that their name would be forgotten--and so it was. I could sometimes feel their frustration--even anger and fear--that their name is never remembered, with the underlying belief: "I am not important." Alan Cohen said, "Today's thoughts are previews of tomorrow's coming attractions."[2]

The consciousnesses from which our intentions arise is important. As important and necessary as the self-help movement has been, it can be excessively narcissistic. It is exciting to see universal concepts like the law of attraction presented to mainstream audiences, though they are often presented in an egotistical and materialistic manner. Focusing on how to change your thoughts only so you can acquire super-sized mansions and attract ever more money misses the point.

Furthermore, visualization and positive thinking can be denial in yet another disguise. Our famous American optimism can be an arrogant refusal to see what is, or an unwillingness to accept our failures. When we focus on what we wish to manifest in the future, we may not be in present time. Again, it can be one more clever way the ego helps us avoid discomfort, trauma, or pain in the body (or problems in the world)--what is here and now--by focusing on where we wish to go.

Be vigilant. Is your consciousness clouded with confusion, humming with thoughts of failure, or flickering with memories of past mistakes? Do you experience background noise of negativity, criticism, and defeat, or consistently bump into walls and limits? Every thought creates. What do you *want* to create? If this moment's thought is not loving, positive, and truthful, if it is not taking you where you want to see yourself and your world, can you switch it?

As we heal and awaken, as we cleanse the energy centers, especially the higher chakras, we become more able to distinguish between our true needs and superficial and egotistical desires and programming. We begin to clear the mind of clutter and confusion, learning to trust and align ourselves. In fact, we come to a point where what we want and what we truly need become the same. We can then begin to filter out the negativity and outer-created images and consciously create the world we truly wish to see.

People doubted Muhammad Yunus, who founded the microcredit-lending Graham Bank in Bangladesh, and went on to win the Nobel-prize for creating bottom-up economic and social development. The bank currently has eight million borrowers, and has empowered women all over the world. When Yunus talks about his goal of completely eliminating global poverty, people laugh, yet he responds, "But when you don't believe something, you can't achieve it. You have to imagine and make that imagination achieveable."[3]

Here is how the creative process works energetically: Ideas initiate in the higher chakras, where the energy, guidance, or inspiration filters down through the crown, and settles into the third eye, the creative landscape of dreams, where we get the actual vision. We can see it--an idea is born! Next, we pass the idea through the throat chakra, where we begin to express our intention: "I want a bike for Christmas!" or sing our song: "Imagine a world at peace . . ."

Then we bring the idea down into the heart, where our initiative begins to form webs of connection into the community and our world. Is it motivated by love? Are we willing to receive this in our life and world? We give our idea *heart*. Next, coming into the third chakra, we create a plan and take physical action, with will power and healthy self-assertion. The second chakra feeds more creative energy, enthusiasm, emotional charge, and ideally pleasure to our creative pursuit--this is why passion is so important to any undertaking or project. Lastly, we root it down into the Earth; we manifest what we have been thinking, imagining, planning, and acting on. The seeds that were originally dropped down from the Universe sprout back up and out into the Earth.

The most important thing is to let go and trust that the Universe will handle the details, often in surprisingly creative ways. For this process to succeed, ideally we must clear any inauthentic intentions, as well as restricting emotions such as fear and guilt. We let go and let the energy flow into that powerful current of appropriate, unattached action, and effortless surrender. What is authentically good for me is good for we. We can change anythng, one image at a time.

This is a profound creative practice of compassionate awareness, and like all spiritual laws, it is essentially simple. Be present. Think love, see love, be love. Can we start now, with this very next thought, image, or word?

෨ Practice Points

- Begin to notice and catch yourself when you are thinking negative thoughts or visualizing failure or disaster. Can you flip the switch?

- Create a collage, vision board, or manifestation map. Gather or clip magazine words, photos, and images that represent the life you wish to create and see, personally and globally. Paste them on a large sheet, and hang them where you can see them daily.

෨ Contemplation: Imagine That

- Get quiet, and take a deep breath. Allow energy to run down through the entire body, down into the Earth. Touch base with your heart center.

- Open your heart, and get in touch with one thing you would like to see on a personal level. More joy? Awakening? Clarity? Healthy relationship?

- Then settle your awareness in the third eye (between and slightly above the eyes). Visualize this happening, like watching a movie.

- Bring awareness into the belly area. Feel passion for your plan!

- Then imagine planting this seed into the Earth and watching it sprout.

- Do the same with a global goal. From the heart, choose something you would like to see or help create in our world. Visualize, and enjoy the creative process.

GRATITUDE

When you go to a garden, do you look at thorns or flowers? Spend more time with roses and jasmine.

- Rumi

Gratitude is the gentle spring rain that nourishes our inner garden, accelerating growth and abundance. If it is true that the universe mirrors our energy, thoughts, and actions, then projecting thanks and appreciation will give us yet more to be grateful for. We will watch our own projected images and joy come back to us.

Jesus, put it simply: "For whoever has, to him more shall be given; and whoever does not have, even what he has shall be taken away from him."[1] While this may not sound fair, it is an impartial and neutral principle of our universe. Our thoughts, words, and actions reverberate through the world like ripples in a pond, enhancing and expanding whatever message we project.

If we are making poverty level income, but manage to shift our thoughts to gratitude and begin visualizing abundant and fruitful ways of living, we will most likely see those changes occur in our life. Conversely, if we inherit fifty million dollars, but continue to dwell on scarcity, we will watch that money dissipate before our eyes.

Undoubtedly, there is plenty to be alarmed about in our world. There are tremendous Earth challenges, political problems, social and health concerns, and countless other human dramas, and it is a challenge to see the cup half full. But there is nothing enlightening about worrying and negativity. We can be informed, that is--formed from within--without losing ourselves in the drama.

Most news coverage does not focus on gratitude, goodness, or good news. Recently a research group analyzed the front pages of the British newspapers, comparing positive versus negative stories. In the seventies, at the peak of the Cold War, there was one positive story for every three negative stories. Thirty years later, there was only one positive story for every seventeen negative stories.[2] We can lay down the newspaper or change the channel.

I like the bumper sticker: wag more, bark less, although I

did a lot more whining than wagging when I was struggling with depression in my forties. Slowly, I managed to begin seeing and appreciating some of the little blessings: my rented room, the few friends I had, my old but economical car, my new pet kitten. As I felt a taste of acceptance, more blessings arrived: more friends, a date or two, and starting a small business. Thus, it became easier to feel gratitude, and eventually greater gifts began to show up in my life: improved health, a successful business, and a growing community of friends. Today, it is not only wise and pragmatic but easier and more natural for me to sit each morning in my meditation and bless each of these areas of my life that were previously less abundant. I can only *imagine* what will happen next!

In the Yoga Sutras, Patanjali discusses the idea of *Santosha*, which might seem radical to us Westerners. Santosha is simply contentment, or seeing the perfection in each of life's precious moments and experiences. Can we feel gratitude for those areas of our life that are *not* going the way we would like? Can we bless the experience of low income, the experience of confusion or depression, the experience of loneliness, or the experience of career/economic/ health woes? This is challenging, but we can trust and accept that *where we are* is first of all impermanent, and secondly, teaching us something. Can we bless it all? I knew I was getting somewhere when I could honestly look back and appreciate the experience and despair of the depression and eating disorder, and all the lessons, people, and inner resources that helped me survive. Life is so rich!

Accompanying this grace of gratitude is the unlimited power we have to do and be and create anything we so choose. By accepting and blessing what we already see, have, and experience in our life, we are able to live more fully right where we are. By envisioning and dreaming, without attachment, we are able to build on the bounty, and create ever more peace, joy, and love in our world.

∞ Practice Points

- Catch yourself when you are grumbling or complaining, and see if you can shift the words, thoughts, or energy to acceptance and appreciation.
- Praise, compliment, and say thank you more often, silently as well as out loud.

Ꮽ Contemplation

- Silently say thank you to each current gift in your life: your next breath, whatever health you enjoy, food, shelter, pets, friends . . .
- Silently acknowledge the challenging areas of your life that you wish to change, and bless each of them. Can you accept or even appreciate what is? What are they teaching you?

BOUNDARIES

In my experience, the way we constantly distort our energy field into our habitual defense system causes more pain and illness in ourselves than any other cause.

- Barbara Ann Brennan

We all have energy fields, or auras, around our bodies, with which we are consciously or unconsciously interacting with our world. Boundary setting is an awareness, ability, or attempt to distinguish or create energetic spaces between us, protect our energy, and avoid negatively affecting one another.

We learn about boundaries and personal space by what is modeled to us, and many of our models are less than exemplary. Many of us push, control, invade, or allow ourselves to be pushed, controlled, or invaded. We soon learn secondary patterns to protect ourselves, some by withdrawing, and others by pushing back (or each at different times). There are countless ways our energy fields interact.

Some specific examples of ignoring or violating personal boundaries are: calling at midnight, talking too much, tailgating, or allowing your dog to bark all night. Examples of more serious or larger scale boundary violations might be burglary, rape, torture, dumping toxic waste, or invading other nations. Areas like Israel and Palestine have been battling over boundaries for decades. Ideally, we align our laws with our commonly agreed boundaries, but this is always imperfect. Is there such a thing as common space? If I am hungry, and someone else has plenty, is it wrong to take an apple off their tree?

Boundaries take their healthiest form when we learn how to become aware and trust ourselves as to what feels right for all involved. As we ground, become more present, and heal old wounds, we find ourselves more clear, neutral, and strong, and less likely to be affected by others' wounds or boundary violations. We have fewer triggers. We are solid yet soft, strong yet yielding. We learn to recognize and let love, support, and healing energy in, but filter out the hate, jealousy, fear, rage, and other harmful energies.

Do you find yourself avoiding social situations because you cannot hold your space? Do you feel your energy drain when you are in certain situations, or do you get a creepy feeling around specific people? Conversely, do you feel your energy rise, and feel uplifted in certain environments or around particular people?

Nonresistance and neutrality help tremendously with setting healthy boundaries. If we are afraid of people or having to set boundaries, we can be sure to attract nothing but people who will test our boundaries! Again, we all interact energetically, so boundaries can be tricky. We all test one another's boundaries, and we all give up our space from time to time. Few of us do this boundary thing "perfectly."

We are constantly adjusting and adapting our energy and boundaries to each situation. Maybe one person needs to be dealt with by patience. Another needs a strong "No!" with a hint of anger behind it. Sometimes we have to leave the scene. If we simply do not want to be around certain people or energies, or we are not yet strong enough to deal with them, the loving choice might be to remove ourselves.

I once went to a conference where the speaker, a famous and brilliant author and teacher, was in an off-putting mood. To me, if felt abusive, with her telling the crowd "You should do this," and "You are so wrong," invalidating and even publicly humiliating the people who were brave enough to offer differing opinions. I thought about standing up to invite a dialogue, but did not feel strong enough for the confrontation in front of hundreds of people. So, I went to the ticket counter, asked for a refund, and left.

Some people simply do not have any sense of setting personal boundaries. They may not even know that this is an option. When they do learn, they sometimes go from no boundaries to iron walls. With experience, we can find a healthy balance. Fortunately, many of life's situations provide great opportunities for practicing boundary setting.

Another time, I was physically hurting from an auto accident and had just come from some very intense and painful bodywork. My energy field felt like a porcupine. Interestingly, I was teaching a workshop on healing that night at the college. Just as we were getting started, a woman sitting next to me--who was obviously very sensitive to energy--got up and changed seats away from me, kindly mentioning that my energy field was disturbing her. She was attentive, honest, and brave enough to take care of herself.

While leaving an environment of discomfort, toxicity, or abuse is sometimes important, we still need to stay in *our* space. Too many of us energetically leave the body to escape. Or, we reach out and try to control and manipulate others, to prevent perceived threats. We literally--usually unconsciously--send out energy chords and connections to others. When we energetically move into another's space, we not only interfere with their life and lessons, we are not "home" to take care of what is going on within us. Ideally our focus is on ourselves and our own energy, not on controlling another's. We can carry this example to the macro level. It is interesting that the United States now has over seven hundred military bases around the world, while we could certainly use some attention and energy back home.

What we put out, in any case, comes back to us. The most important thing in setting healthy boundaries is healing ourselves and staying present, connected to our inner energy source. Breathe deeply, and be fully alive and aware in your body and feelings. The heart knows what to do.

Sometimes I will give darshan (healing embrace) to 40,000 people, sitting for 24 hours straight. Even what is considered a big crowd in America is like a vacation for me. I am able to do this because I realize that I am one with the Supreme Self--the main current supply, and therefore I'm not like a battery that needs to be constantly recharged.[1]

- Amma

⌘ **Practice Points**

* During interactions, what happens to your grounding, your breathing, and your emotions?
* Notice how you feel around certain people or situations. Do you let others into your "space" easily, or do you move into their "space"?

⌘ **Contemplation**

* Reflect on how you might respond to each of these situations with healthy boundaries? 1) returning a product at a store where they refuse to give a refund, 2) someone comes by at midnight, or 3) someone is asking for too many favors.
* Generally, how would you like to respond to life's situations with regards to boundaries?

DO UNTO OTHERS

And in the end, the love you take, is equal to the love you make.
- The Beatles

It is fitting that these are the last words of the last song recorded by the Beatles--"The End" on the Abbey Road album. Treating others more kindly may smooth out our own roads ahead.

One day in 2008, I was driving when I heard a honk from the car in the lane to my left. Turning, I was astonished to see a driver, perhaps 40ish, staring aggressively and pointing one of his fingers at me. It took me a moment to realize that he had seen my *Stop the Iraq War* sticker and clearly disagreed, and was trying to start another war. Rather than retaliate as I often would, I smiled sincerely, and showed him a couple fingers of my own--the peace sign--and I saw a slightly stunned smile crease his face.

Ending war begins in our own heart. If I know that I am you and you are me, would I hurt you? Would the liver attack the kidney? The head make war on the heart? Ironically, this is what is happening with our immune systems of late, with parts of our own bodies apparently doing battle with each other. Perhaps we are internalizing our misunderstandings, a microcosm for a world at war with itself, seeing enemies everywhere, inside and out.

We live on a rapidly-changing planet, and until we further our growth and evolution, we need rules or signposts along the way. There is no guideline more useful than the Golden Rule offered to us by Jesus: "So in everything, do to others what you would have them do to you . . ."[1] Here we have the perfect antidote for boundary challenges: treating others how we would like to be treated. Yet loving our neighbor goes beyond a narcissistic giving-to-get. As we awaken, we simply give and love because it is a natural expression of who we are. Jon Kabbat Zinn said, "At the deepest level there is no giver, no gift, and no recipient . . . only the universe rearranging itself."[2]

One day I was at a Seattle fruit and veggie stand, waiting in line to pay. When the clerk mentioned my total, about $4.50, I reached for my wallet but realized it was sitting at home. Feeling silly, I apologized to the clerk and I turned to leave. But a woman in line behind me calmly said, "I'll get it," and quietly paid my bill.

When we fall into separation, we often see our neighbors as enemies rather than another aspect of ourselves. And we cannot separate this message from the political arena. When we make war on another country, or sabotage their electoral process, or support an undemocratic coup, we are inviting the same actions towards our nation. When we call a nation evil, and refuse to communicate, we are cutting off a part of ourselves. There is no other.

Dr. Ihaleakala Hew Len, PhD, offers this wonderful Ho'oponopono prayer: "I love you. I am sorry. Please forgive me (for whatever is going on in me that I perceive the world to be this certain way). Thank you".[3] Ho'oponopono is a Hawaiian word for a form of community and personal therapy or prayer that focuses on healing and forgiveness through taking complete responsibility for one's thoughts. The next time you judge or are angry with someone (or yourself), try silently saying this, and see how it feels: *I love you. I am sorry. Please forgive me. Thank you.* Again, *they* don't need to change--we do.

When we see someone having a bad day, can we not hold

a space of empathy? Furthermore, when we encounter what we perceive as evil or hateful people, can we not evoke even more kindness, knowing that they may be having a bad life?!

Can we trust that Jesus, the Buddha, and other teachers knew what they were talking about? Can we try loving our neighbor, today? Again, we need not do it to change others, but to change ourselves and to ease our own heart. Amazingly, it does change others as well. Rather than enhance their pain, it reflects and encourages their truest nature.

෨ Practice Points

- Without trying to change others, try sending compassionate thoughts, a smile, or lending a helping hand. Notice how this makes you feel: vulnerable? joyful? free?
- If you have trouble with this, can you fake it until you make it more genuine?

෨ Contemplation

- Breathe. Without guilt or pride, reflect on what energy and emotion you have been putting out into the world and into your relationships. Make peace with the past.
- Visualize how you would like to begin treating the world. In particular, is there someone you toward whom would like to be more kind and loving?
- Silently send them compassion and say, "I love you, I am sorry. Please forgive me. Thank you."

SIMPLICITY

If your mind isn't clouded by unnecessary things, this is the best season of your life.
 - Wu-men

I have heard that a good speech or sermon has a good opener, a good finish, and very little in between. Keep it simple and short.

Simple and short are actually richer and more satisfying. The growing simplicity movement is not about suffering or sacrificing as much as releasing what is complex and superfluous. It is about making time and space for what is meaningful and vital to feeling genuinely fulfilled.

On a physical level, have you ever downsized and uncluttered a space, home or office? How does it feel when you give some unessential item away to a friend or thrift store? Does it feel cathartic and liberating?

I had a personal experience with simplicity on my first extended trip outside the U.S. I began an eight month trip to Australia, New Zealand, and Indonesia with a fifty pound backpack, but soon realized I could do with less, much less. Soon I was shedding shirts, gadgets, and knick-knacks by about a pound a week. By the time I got to Indonesia, several months into the trip, my pack had shrunk down to about a third of its original weight. Not only was my backpack feeling lighter with every pound purged, but my own heart grew less dense and more at ease.

Sitting Bull recognized the ways of the white man over 100 years ago: "The love of possessions is a disease among them."[1] Nowadays, with yoga-mania, one can spend hundreds of dollars on trendy gear and attire, but none of this will get us closer to our God. In my classes, we use very few props; there is something about the simplicity of yoga that gives me great pleasure. There are even nude yoga classes in some areas now--not much yoga gear needed here!

We Americans are learning about downsizing and simplifying. For years, the homes were literally less green: while the home sizes increased, the green and garden space around them diminished. The average American home in 1950 was around 1,000 square feet, but by 2005, it was up to 2,500, often with three or four bathrooms. Perhaps we began to realize that bigger homes do not necessarily make us more happy. The good news is that by 2008 people were starting to build smaller homes again, and were creating more garden space.

Helen Keller said, "To me a lush carpet of pine needles or spongy grass is more welcome than the most luxurious Persian rug."[2] Some of us feel that those with the most toys do not win.

We end up constantly stressed, working harder to pay the bills, often spending our weekends fixing our many gadgets. We often lose more than we gain. The marketers have magically created needs out of items previously unheard of. Who had a cell phone or an iPod ten years ago, or even a television one hundred years ago? At first it is challenging to step back and say whoa, is this what I really want or need?

Again, practicing presence is key. The cycle of busyness unwinds as we learn to step out of it and take a deep breath. Every pause in the momentum of madness provides a glimpse of sanity and out of this silence comes the peace of who we already are. We begin to sense what is real, what is important. We connect in community and the ego loses its need for outdoing the neighbors, or impressing others with our packed schedule or loud cell phone conversations. We make time for laughter, connection, and nature: things that feed rather than shatter the soul.

That is enough for this topic; let's keep it simple and short.

Ꮹ Practice Points

- If you haven't used it in a year, give it away or recycle it. Have a give-away or trade party, or a garage sale.
- Turn off the TV except for nourishing or educational programs.
- Work close to home, and walk or ride a bike when possible.
- Make time for what is important to you: prayer, relationships, hobbies, volunteering, nature, fitness, music . . .
- Practice all this with a spirit of joy and abundance.

Ꮹ Contemplation

- Breathe easily but deeply. Without straining, notice and enjoy the slight pause at the end of the out breath, just before the in breath.

SACRED SPACE

Never go to a doctor whose office plants have died.
- Erma Bombeck

Every space, in truth, is sacred; no place is "better" than any other place. How can one aspect or manifestation of the Divine be superior to any other?

There are places, though, where the earthly energy vibration or frequency is higher, more natural, more potent. In the United States, Sedona, Arizona is reportedly one such spot. Hawaii has a magical aliveness. The California Redwoods have a special energy, as does the Olympic Rainforest in Washington State.

Does this mean we need to fly across the country or around the world to find sacred space? Perhaps not. Is there a virgin forest in your area, a colorful desert, or a pristine lake or river? How about a simple park with greenery, or even your own garden? Maybe you know a particular teahouse, yoga studio, community center, or church. If you do not know of any, create one--perhaps even in your own home. On a community, national, and global level, we can help create or preserve sacred space by actively supporting the preservation of our wild lands and green zones. By saving nature we are actually saving ourselves.

Most of us know that nature nourishes, balances, and enlivens. Forests, parks, and even potted plants foster people's sense of kindness, health, happiness, and community. Natural environments--the precious few that remain--feed *our* very nature. The Earth's sacred pulse alleviates emotional angst, calms the mind, and soothes the soul. Natural environments still beat to the ancient rhythms of the Earth, vibrating energetically to a tempo that matches our deepest nature, previous to the array of modern energies and toxins that bombard, bruise, and batter our senses twenty-four hours a day.

It is interesting that as we moved away from nature, we became unwell. From 1873 to 1923 the number of hospitals in the U.S. increased 3,800 percent.[1] The mysterious Georgia Guide Stones advise us, and even repeat the last words: "Be not a cancer on the earth. Leave room for nature. Leave room for nature." A reporter once asked Gandhi what he thought about Western civilization, to which he replied, "It would be a good idea."[2]

The modern world draws us up into our heads, because there is more need to think, plan, and calculate. Our primordial tools of intuition and instincts are less valued, resulting in disembodiment and disconnect from the critical and profoundly healing arena of sensual experience. In our hardened world, there is a reason we shut down our senses: we do not want to see the turmoil, hear the noise, smell the exhaust fumes, or feel the frenzied energy. We sense the nonsense, so we close down. We grow so accustomed to the density, noise, and angst of our refined world that we simply forget our own nature.

We've recently added the term "nature deficit disorder" to describe the negative side effects of living in our modern society. When we are in the wilds, it is easy and natural to return to our senses; we often like what we hear, smell, see, and feel. Although I am a fairly anxious person, it takes but a few hours in nature to calm me down, and an overnight backpack trip really balances and enlivens my energy system. No expensive therapy or support groups are needed--just the free and generous community of trees and water and rocks. Anne Frank said, "The best remedy for those who are afraid, lonely, or unhappy is to go outside, somewhere they can be quiet, alone with the heavens, nature, and God."[3]

Many of us--especially during the gray winters here in the Pacific Northwest--do not get sufficient sunlight to create enough vitamin D. I have heard that in certain indigenous communities in South America, an imbalanced person is sat by a river until well-being is restored. Similarly, in Mexico, when someone goes crazy or gets out of whack, they sit the person against a tree until the person feels grounded again.

It is only a sign of our disconnect from reality when we cannot distinguish between an old growth and a second- or third-growth forest. With attention, we can *feel* the difference. I went on a couple of hikes in recent years that crossed through clear cut areas and was amazed at the sad, heavy, dead energy. Interestingly, I experienced headaches after both those hikes, which I had never experienced on previous hikes. It is simply untrue that forests and wild lands quickly recover. As capable as nature is, it may take hundreds or thousands of years for her to balance and rebuild her intricate web of relations and living communities.

Of course, planting trees and plants tremendously shifts the energy, as well as providing oxygen, shade, beauty, noise buffers, and homes for our fellow critters. The gray world of pavement is such a deprivation for all of us--adults and children. Concrete hardens our heart, while rocks ground us. Skyscrapers diminish us into timidity, while ancient trees help us stand strong and tall.

Gandhi said, "To forget how to dig the Earth and to tend the soil is to forget ourselves."[4] One reason for our deep fear and anxiety is our disconnect with the Earth and the very food we eat. Getting back into the garden and growing our own groceries is healing and empowering. We so need the sacred Earth beneath our feet, and the dirt between our toes and fingers.

We can still try to sense the holy even in the most mundane, material manifestations. Ultimately, that which is most sacred is that which is closest to nature. Make time for the natural world, which literally returns us to our roots, realigns us to the rhythms of the Earth, and connects us to what is present and alive. And we can always visit and know that deepest divinity within ourselves. Wherever we go, there is the sacred.

Look deep into nature, and then you will understand everything better.[5]
- Albert Einstein

ᱛᱺ Practice Points

- Next time you are feeling stressed, afraid, or confused, make time for a park walk or nature visit. Notice how you feel.
- Do your best to make every place you visit "sacred." See its beauty. Add a special touch. How might you create sacred space in and around your home?

ᱛᱺ Contemplation: Sacred Space

- Wherever you presently are--during this meditation--make it sacred and safe: breathe, ground, and lighten up. Feel the sacred, here, now.
- Picture yourself in the most safe and sacred natural setting you can imagine. It may be a real, beautiful location you have been to, or simply use your imagination.
- Breathe deeply and take in the healing energy of that place. Take it into your very cells, and let it cleanse all the fear and anxiety from your body.

PART FIVE: PEACE WITH PAIN

EARTH CHALLENGES

There is a way that nature speaks, that land speaks. Most of the time we are simply not patient enough, quiet enough, to pay attention to the story.
 - Linda Hogan

One winter evening in 2007, alarmingly strong winds belted our Pacific Northwest region, blowing shakes off many roofs, and knocking power out of much of the Seattle area. I got a disquieting feeling that this was not just some odd storm, but something eerily significant, a sign of global climate changes. I asked my then-partner Laura, "Am I paranoid or does something feel out of whack, as if the Earth is shouting to get our attention?" A few minutes later Laura called me downstairs to see what had happened to our Earth flag on the front porch: the wind had blown the Earth out of middle of the flag.

Many ancient and indigenous groups have written or warned about the dramatic changes that would happen on planet Earth, culminating around this very time. Author Neale Donald Walsch says, "We are seeing the beginnings of what I call The Shift right now as we witness the wholesale rearrangement of our planet's economics, its politics, its religions . . ."[1] It is both an exhilarating and terrifying time to be alive!

The suggestions offered in this book may be helpful in

handling these planetary changes that are *now* occurring. We can ground, breathe deeply, pay attention, build community, and be willing to see things with new eyes. That we have *not* been doing these things may be one reason for the Earth challenges. The solutions will not come only from thinking and the intellect, but from the silence of the heart, and the intelligence of the Earth and Universe itself.

It has been said that if we do not take care of the Earth, the Earth will take care of us! On some level, we know that we humans have become like fleas that the Earth is scratching and desperately trying to remove. Some speak of "Nature's Fury,"and the "Raging Earth," but there is nothing personal about the intense and often destructive winds and waves that are striking many parts of our world. The Earth is simply using all its tools--water, wind, temperature, and vibration--to purify and purge itself, and we are being shaken from our sleep and comfort zone.

Why have we been so slow to wake up and respond to the Earth changes? Frogs, when placed in a pot of hot water, will waste no time in bounding out of harm's way. But set in cold water that is slowly heated, they will allow themselves to cook. Perhaps we have numbed ourselves and contaminated our nest so steadily that we have forgotten what a vibrant, natural environment would look and feel like. I would guess that if we plucked a Native American from her home a thousand years ago and placed her in a big American city today, she would run for the woods!

The reasons for our mistreatment of the Earth are many, but stem from our state of consciousness. As we disconnected from our emotions, body, and the bigger body Earth, and identified with ego, we lost our spiritual sustenance. We sought comfort and pleasure in material comforts, like anchoring ourselves to the wrong mooring.

The mainstream media refuses to explore the deepest issues. We somehow convince ourselves that more weapons make us safer. We casually talk about clean coal and nuclear power as safe and sustainable energies. We bury nuclear waste along with our emotions, pretending and hoping they will never surface. Is it a coincidence that the 15 hottest years on record occurred since 1991? Is it okay to lose a third of the Arctic ice in just the last 30 years?

There are naysayers who deny an Earth problem, or argue that we must move slowly. But if something is wrong, it needs to change. If someone is hurting a child, do we show patience? No--we stop the abuse now.

We have already seen how emotions can be pointing to something essential. Personally, I do not *feel* good when I take the garbage out each week, or when I drive my car. I *feel ashamed* when I hear that we Americans consume a disproportionate share of the world's resources while creating enormous amounts of carbon dioxide and toxic waste. I *feel sad, scared, and angry* hearing that one third of the Earth's animal and plant species are now facing extinction.[2] Our disembodied denial of honest emotional responses has us at the brink of self-destruction. Deepak Chopra says, "The underlying question comes down to this: Are we causing earth changes? The spiritual answer is, of course we are, because Mother Nature is disturbed by our lack of love and respect for her."[3]

Personally, I *feel* better when I ride my bicycle, or when I hang my clothes on the line, or mow my little lawn with my quiet, stink-free human-powered mower. I *enjoy* growing food in our neighborhood community garden. It *feels* right printing this book using the most "green," recycled paper available. Granted, these are small things, but small things matter. Change can be stressful, but with teamwork and bold action, we can go from feeling alone, ashamed, and afraid to feeling connected, empowered, and alive.

No one knows for sure what will happen in 2012 or thereabouts. The ancients and many modern scientists seem to agree that this is a very rare alignment, a precession of the equinoxes--that the Mayans and others say happens only once every 26,000 years. Some, including the Mayans, and Edgar Cayce in the 1930s, predicted that this event would reverse the north and south poles and perhaps immerse the Earth in darkness for several days. There is much speculation and trepidation, but the changing energies are certainly affecting our stress and depression rates, and shaking the foundations of our social, political, economic, and other systems. But perhaps some of this is essentially out of our hands. What we certainly *can* do, however, is our inner healing work so we can be as emotionally, spiritually, and physically ready as possible for this tremendous shift.

Human beings can be wise, compassionate, creative, and constructive, and when we motivate ourselves, we can move quite fast. Every year we learn about more Earth-, energy-, and life-saving discoveries and innovations utilizing solar, wind, tidal, geothermal, and algae to provide clean energy. Let us remember that we are truly capable of miracles. When we work together, we can rock this world, but to a healing beat.

The word apocalypse has Greek origins that actually translate as "lifting of the veil," or "revelation." We are awakening to see the oneness and interconnectedness, and understanding that what we call the "environment" is truly our extended body or energy field.

Our world is changing. We can surrender to the falling apart, while preparing to create something profoundly more beautiful, and infinitely more satisfying and sustainable. We are so blessed to be here on Earth during this historic and magnificent shifting of global consciousness.

Do not be afraid. Let the morning come. Let the dawn come. May the people find peace and be happy.[4]
- Don Alejandro Cirilo Perez

ᙀ Practice Points

- Notice how you feel when you live in ways that may be harming our planet.
- Notice how you feel when you connect with your community, and live in ways that are more simple, green, and sustainable.

ᙀ Contemplation: Listening to Mother Earth

- Feel your feet, your connection with the Earth. Breathe deeply and listen. What is the Earth saying?
- How does your body feel about what is going on today on Earth? Listen and respond to your own body and emotional needs and see if this actually helps the bigger body Earth as well.

RADICAL RESPONSIBILITY

The pollution of the planet is only an outward reflection of an inner psychic pollution: millions of unconscious individuals not taking responsibility for their inner space.

- Eckhart Tolle

Responsible means *able to respond, answerable for, trustworthy.* Most of us would probably say we are responsible. But it is often the wrong response!

Frequently, we are tempted to take responsibility for others, as in changing or healing them. As a peace activist, I know this one quite well. To me, doing human rights work in Central America actually seemed easier than doing the inner work, taking responsibility for myself. My ego loved focusing on educating *others* and urging shifts in U.S. policy. That somehow seemed more doable or important than taking responsibility for my own pain, my own mind, and my own unloving thoughts.

While Gandhi was in prison, a man wrote to him asking how he could help heal their country, to which Gandhi replied: "Do not burden yourself with the responsibility of emancipating the country. Emancipate yourself, this burden is good enough. Begin applying all principles to your life, considering that you are India. In this rests the salvation of your soul. In this rests the salvation of India."[1]

We may say, "If I could just change that other person (or country), my life will be better. If they would change, I would be happy." Again, when we focus our energy on others, rather than ourselves, we interrupt their growth process, and hinder our own at the same time. We are not home taking care of our self.

But coming home, taking radical responsibility for our own issues, focusing on what we can do differently in our own lives, is scary work. The ego likes to be right; humility is not its forte. The only thing the ego likes to take responsibility for is that which it judges as good or praiseworthy. There is a story of a man who leaves late for an important appointment, and then upon arrival, can't find a parking spot. Cussing the situation, he shouts out, "God, find me a parking space and I promise I'll be more responsible!" Instantly, he sees a spot open up, and says, "Never mind God, I found one."

Accepting and taking an honest, compassionate, and radical responsibility--without judgment for self or others--heals our world and our selves. When we deny, or blame someone else, we simply hand over our power. Are we responsible for what we have created, and for our experience here on Earth at this time? Or, did we just end up here, by fate, with no say in the matter? Or, perhaps it's someone else's fault: God, our parents, or the government. When you stop seeing yourself as a helpless victim of a cruel and senseless world, then you can reclaim the power you used in creating it, and use that same power to create anew.

As we hold *ourselves* responsible, however, we must also hold our own government, banks, and other institutions responsible. We the American people are often resented more than represented, and our system is less a democracy than plutocracy--rule by the elite. While about one percent of Americans were millionaires in 2009, forty-four percent of our members of Congress--or 237 members--were millionaires.[2] In recent years, we have not had a truly free and fair market, but a crooked, crony, corporate capitalism, which, for example, rewards the dirty industries of oil, coal, and nuclear power with billions of dollars in subsidies each year. The invisible hand that manages the market is often not an open hand of fairness but a closed fist of greed. All this comes at a cost. Mayan elder don Alejandro Cirilo Perez warns, "There will be grave occurrences on the face of the Earth. We won't be able to buy the sun, the water, the air."[3]

Yet each and every one of us needs to take responsibility for our nation's senselessness and yes, even insanity. We kill people to prove that killing is wrong. We terrorize people to fight terror. We build and drop bombs to punish others for having bombs--which we often sell them, since the U.S. is the world's biggest arms dealer. We refuse to see the true costs of our decisions and policies.

Returning to the events of September 11th, in the same way, forgiveness was ruled out because it was deemed treasonous to discuss any responsibility for our part in what occurred. Of course, bringing the guilty parties to justice is important. But it was, and is, political suicide to suggest that, along with physically securing our homeland, we could take a critical look at our government's policies, our way of life, and our treatment of other peoples and the Earth itself. Karma waves no flag. When we change ourselves now, we change what happens to us in the future.

Personal healing is global healing. When we see the problems of this world as our own, as something we collectively create, then we can help heal them. On the other hand, we can release our narrow, anthropocentric focus and remember that it is not all about humans. The Earth will probably survive, even if many of us are removed.

Yes, there are present dangers and threats in this world, but it takes great presence, responsibility, courage, and vision to understand that the problem is in our own minds. And when we change our mind, we change the world. There is a Chinese proverb: *When one leaf trembles, the whole bough moves.*

෨ Practice Points

- Practice taking compassionate, radical responsibility for your thoughts and actions.

෨ Contemplation: Radical Responsibility

- Take a deep breath. Reflect: How is your life affecting the whole? In what ways have you been responsible? In what ways have you been irresponsible?
- How can you take radical responsibility for yourself, your energy, and your life?

MAKE USE OF SUFFERING

You desire to know the art of living, my friend? It is contained in one phrase: make use of suffering.
- Henri-Frédéric Amiel

The great yogi Krishnamacharya would say, "Thank God for *duhkha*"[1] (suffering), which he considered the unavoidable motivation for our yoga or spiritual practice. In other words, suffering gets our attention, invites us to delve deeper, beneath the mundane and beyond the illusions. Accept suffering, and it becomes your teacher, ally, and perhaps even your friend.

Henry David Thoreau said, "The mass of men lead lives of quiet desperation."[2] The Buddha said that life is suffering, and certainly none of us escapes it. For years the Buddha searched and struggled for meaning, and Jesus went through hell to show us heaven. All of us have our dark night of the soul, *if we are lucky*. If we embrace it, we can transform its richness, so we do not go through life half-alive. Like the beautiful lotus flower, which arises from the dirtiest waters, we can emerge purified from our pain with evermore depth and dignity.

Perhaps I am just jealous, but those who go through life smoothly, raised in functional families (there *are* some aren't there?), not detouring into the deepest darkness, just may be missing out on life's richness. If you only experience easiness and abundance in your life, you may be pleasant and assured, but possibly shallow and bored. Without darkness, how can we know light? The mid-life crisis is really a mid-life opportunity, for it is inviting us out of mediocrity and into wholeness and greatness. As spiritual teacher Michael Mirdad says, ". . . in truth, the Soul Transformation Process (and its extreme version known as the "dark night of the soul") is the most powerful initiatory process known to mankind."[3]

We already mentioned that according to the Yoga Sutras, ignorance is considered the root of all suffering. This fundamental confusion about the nature of our deepest reality and interconnectedness often underlies all downstream suffering: ego-identification, fear, guilt, worry, scarcity thinking, attachment (to things, people, outcomes, and beliefs), and aversion (again, to things, people, outcomes, and beliefs).

Let me add here that ego is not *bad*, as everything in this world has a place. Although at times I've criticized the ego harshly in this book, let me be clear: it is all good and it's all God. Ego gives us the ability to have the experience of individual separation, to identify our self in this world. Ego may help us understand the nature of suffering!

We create problems, however, when we remain limited to ego-alignment. In *Meditation For Dummies*, Stephan Bodian says, "The great meditative traditions teach that the root cause of suffering and stress, which gives rise to your stories, is the belief that you're inherently separate--from others, from the rest of life, and from being itself."[4] The war is over when we finally understand that you are me and I am you and We are the one Reality. Then we can put down our weapons, whose barrels really point both ways. As already mentioned, why would one part of itself fight another?

One of my college yoga students wrote, "I dwell on my past mistakes and repeatedly beat myself up over them." What this does is continue the karma-samskara cycle of suffering. By fighting and judging ourselves or the pain, we create yet another wounding that must play itself out with further suffering.

There is a saying in Spanish, "No hay mal que por bien no venga" (good always arises from the bad.) Victor Frankl in his wonderful book, *Man's Search for Meaning*, decided to make use of his suffering in the concentration camps. He made a commitment to write about his experience, to share his life's lessons, and his suffering served a purpose. We can find meaning and passion in life's pain, and it's up to each of us to decide that meaning.

We suffer when we resist and fight what is, or when we withhold ourselves from life. When we lock the lid on our joy and love--or our fear and anxiety--we are not allowing life to flow through us. And there is a space within us beyond the suffering. If we can breathe deeply and trust, we can access this place, decide that we are here on Earth for a reason, that our human challenges are not trite or unfair or without reason. We can invent a reason! At the very least, it will ease the struggle, the madness, and the blame. It might even change our world.

At any rate, can we remember that everything in this world, including suffering, is temporary? For those of us who feel that we got the worst incarnation, we can think--or thank--again. You may not always get what you want, but you always get what you need.

Stressed spelled backwards is *desserts*, so always look for the goodies. Stress and suffering can be our greatest teachers, providing fuel and incentive for greater growth in consciousness. We can learn empathy and compassion. We can share and teach what we have experienced, and we can appreciate the loveliness and grace of easier moments.

ᙦ Practice Points

• As you go through your day, notice sources of suffering. Experiment with breathing deeply, a breath of compassion for self and others.

ᙦ Contemplation: Seeds of Awakening

• Breathe. Reflect on any seeds of suffering in your life: attachment, aversion, ego identification, fear, or ignorance.

• Can you accept these seeds as they are for the moment? Can you feel compassion for your imperfect human self? Is it possible to use pain and suffering as seeds for awakening?

LEARN FROM FAILURE AND CHALLENGE

I've failed my way to success.
- Thomas Edison

Here, we will expand on the goal of learning from suffering to embracing all of life's challenges and failings. None of us humans go through an entire life--or day--without making a mistake or failing at something. All of us have hit walls, pain, or challenges, some of which may feel insurmountable.

How quick is the ego to label circumstances, events, and results as good or bad, success or failure! If we hold the view that failure, mistakes, and challenges should be avoided or eliminated, we are out of touch with reality. Life is messy, but there is perfection in failure and challenge. Life's speed bumps can either derail us or cause us to pause, and elevate us to a higher perspective and understanding.

Crises are rich with opportunity. Franklin Delano Roosevelt, considered one of America's greatest Presidents, used the chaos of the Great Depression to initiate the New Deal and some of the most significant legislation ever, including the Social Security System, the Works Progress Administration, and the Civilian Conservation Corps. President Barack Obama commented during the deepening recession in February of 2008 that the moment "is full of peril but full of possibility."[1] Challenge invites the best in us.

We may not consciously choose all of life's dramas, tests, and failings. When you ride your bike or go hiking, you might not purposely select the steepest route, but the inevitable hills you climb may deepen your breath, quicken the heart, and help you discover something about yourself. How can we know and appreciate downhill ease and success without uphill climbs and challenge? How can we appreciate the view from the highest mountain without crossing through the lowest valley?

Basketball star Michael Jordan was initially cut from his first high school team! He now says, "I've missed more than 9,000 shots in my career. I've lost almost 300 games. Twenty-six times, I've been trusted to take the game-winning shot, and missed. I've failed over and over and over again in my life--and that is why I succeed."[2]

Throughout most of my life, when confronted with strife, I often whined, withered, blamed, or raged, and did not like my own company. I would feel puny, powerless, and immobilized by my weakness. I was so jealous yet impressed by those people who seemed to bounce back easily and effortlessly from adversity and problems. Did they even have any problems? How did they do that?

One morning, I walked out of my house, only to see an empty space where my car had been parked. I immediately recalled that my insurance did not cover the stolen car, and I knew I could not afford another one. Predictably, I felt the start of a whining and moping stage. This time, however, I cut it short. I sent out an email to my friends asking for help, and the energy quickly shifted. One friend lent me a spare car, while another well-off friend sent a check to help cover some of the loss. Another dropped off a toy car with a note saying "Car-ma: you will be okay." The time without a car also helped me consider my attachment to cars. Then two weeks later, the police found my car and another friend gave me a ride to pick it up. I learned to ask for help--which in the past had been a very uncomfortable thing--and rather than feeling victimized, I came out empowered by the whole event.

The journey to healing old patterns and beliefs is so rich and rewarding. Jack Kornfield says, "To undertake a genuine spiritual path is not to avoid difficulties but to learn the art of making mistakes wakefully, to bring to them the transformative power of our heart...The basic principle of spiritual life is that our problems become the very place to discover wisdom and love."[3]

For many of us, a dysfunctional family of origin or an imperfect childhood was our greatest challenge, and the wounds endured may still create present day suffering. Can we be brave enough, though, to question old assumptions and beliefs? What if we accept that each of us had the perfect mother and father or childhood for what we needed to experience and learn here on Earth in this lifetime--what our personal karma called forth? Family relationships can be treasure chests of lessons.

The end of an intimate relationship can be stressful, but perhaps not as dramatic as we make it. You may fall apart, believe you have failed or that you will never again find true love. But as Rumi said, "You moan, 'She left me.' 'He left me.' Twenty more will come."[4] We can learn from every one of life's precious relationships, and judge them more on the lessons and joy rather than the duration or challenges.

Many of us have challenges that feel much bigger than stolen cars and broken romances. Life can be trying, and sometimes the best we can do is just accept and pray or ask for guidance, help, and understanding. The point is, can we trust that the universe has more vision than any of us humans? Can we learn from our mistakes and build on what we have experienced? We can crawl out from beneath our broken hearts and failed romances, dust ourselves off from our slayings by critics, and arise the wiser for it.

There is a Zen saying: "The snow falls, each flake in its appropriate place." When we make peace with the present moment, when we move with the intelligence of trust and confidence, nothing can shake us from our roots and our core connection with Spirit.

⊚ **Practice Points**

- Notice how you react or respond when something does not go your way, or when you "fail," or make a mistake. Breathe deeply, and simply be present to your feelings. Allow a breath of compassion.

⊚ **Contemplation: Lessons from Challenge**

- Look back on things you saw as horrible failures, bad luck, mistakes, or overwhelming challenges. Are there any gifts or lessons you received from these experiences?
- Breathe acceptance for what is, and what has been. What are you currently challenged with? What is it teaching you? How can you accept it and overcome it?

RELATIONSHIPS AS MIRRORS

But when you make peace with yourself, the world will mirror back that same level of peace.
- Debbie Ford

Do you bless or curse your relationship "mirrors"? Although not every human encounter feels particularly comfortable, every relationship does offer an opportunity for growth, healing, and self-discovery.

I once had a housemate, a young fellow of perhaps twenty-three; I'll call him Ben. Having endured an apparently painful and abusive youth, Ben was regularly carrying a shadow of rage. One day, he left the house, and immediately came across another young man walking down the sidewalk. They took one look at each other, something sparked, and the other fellow lunged at Ben and punched him in the face. The attack quickly triggered Ben's own rage, helping him overcome--and pummel--the equally surprised attacker.

A coincidental encounter? Nope. We tend to attract who we are. Ben's energy field of pain and rage triggered the attack from the other angry young man. They looked each other in the eye, and did not like what they saw, for they saw themselves.

Pain--as any energy--needs movement and release. If you do not find the space and focus to feel and express what is within you, you'll find ways to get your own attention. If you have a backlog, this is not always pleasant. It is important to see that this sidewalk encounter was in fact necessary, as the denied pain-bubble had to burst. Ideally we find ways to express this energy safely before we explode.

Relationships can be frustrating precisely because they are mirroring back what we need to see and know about ourselves. Anyone who triggers us is revealing the most pressing priority to be faced and healed. Generally, the more frequently a type of person appears in your life, the more you want to pay attention. If you wonder and whine about the selfish people who keep showing up in your life, you might want to look at your own selfishness. If a frightened person rubs you the wrong way, perhaps you have some fear to deal with. If you are knocked off center by anxious people, you may need to explore your own stress level. The flaws we see in others may in fact be our own.

The reverse can also be true. If a person bugs us because they talk too much, we may need to speak up a bit more. If we are jealous at someone's ability to handle life's challenges, we might want to explore our own power issues. Often someone takes on the form of a hero. We admire them greatly, for they are showing us an aspect of ourselves we have not yet developed, allowed, or recognized. Pay careful attention, for gifts abound.

The intensity of the trigger--whether it is a person or event--correlates directly with the depth of our denial. Conversely, the depth of the potential lesson and healing increases with our biggest bumps and challenging confrontations. We are subconsciously shouting for our own attention. We often judge others rather than thank our mirror and face our own denied energy, whether pain or passion.

The deeper we go with our growth and evolution, the more we will attract resistance against us until we do the deepest inner work to heal all that is incompatible with love. The key is to decide for ourselves the significance of life's encounters. We are making this whole game up ourselves, and we have the power to whine or win. Rather than resist our reflections, we can decide that every relationship--in fact everything life offers--holds a gift. What we judge in others is often simply a projection--we see it more clearly in others than ourselves at that point. Jesus put it clearly, "You hypocrite, first take the log out of your own eye, and then you will see clearly to take the speck out of your brother's eye."[1]

The Dalai Lama reportedly never enters a meeting with an adversary without first visualizing himself in that person's shoes. The Yoga Sutras, similar to Buddhism, invite us to compassion and equanimity in our relationships. Sutra 1.33 translates something like this: "undisturbed calmness of mind is attained by cultivating friendliness toward the happy, compassion for the unhappy, joyfulness towards those who are successful, and neutrality towards evil." You keep your heart open. Rather than protect your fragile self-image by judging and seeing "other," you come to see that there is only one universe shining a light on everything that needs attention.

When we lose ourselves in this Earthly reality (or falsity), and descend into the delusion and drama, we may forget that the healing and guidance we so desperately prayed for has arrived! The angels and teachers we have sought may initially be hard to recognize, appearing as thieves and rapists, liars and cheats. If we forget that we have indeed invited and created every encounter, every experience, to help us know and grow, then we may paint ourselves as victims, rather than brave and powerful participants in the creative process. So can we accept our own gifts? Can we praise our ingenuity? Can we celebrate and recognize that we magically and masterfully draw to us all the people, events, and situations we choose to assist us on our evolutionary path?

Be gentle with yourself, for this is brave and holy work. The shift occurs, with its accompanying sense of freedom, when we realize that we are all Divine Beings imperfectly struggling in human form with our pain, our grief, our resentment, and our confusion. With humility, we can bless, thank, and learn from our mirrors. Eventually we will like what we see reflected back at us.

ᏔᏜ Practice Points

- Pay close attention whenever someone triggers you: what is this telling you about *yourself*? What needs to be seen, accepted, and healed?

◎ Contemplation: Shadow Reflections

* Breathe deeply. Look at three people who push your buttons. What is the main characteristic about them that bugs you? Ask yourself: Do I have these traits? Have I ever had them? Or do I do the opposite out of judgment and resistance to those traits?

MAKING PEACE WITH PAIN

We cannot heal what we cannot feel.
- John Bradshaw

If you are human, you know pain. In fact, there is a chance you are feeling some degree of pain right this moment, be it physical, emotional, or of the soul. Dealing with acute or chronic pain is one of our greatest human challenges.

To have any chance of relieving pain, we first need to acknowledge it, feel it, and accept it. Many of us have been taught--and indeed it is intuitive--to move away from pain. Our bodies know this: when our finger touches something hot, we withdraw. Many new age thinkers teach "feel good" positive thinking and affirmations, and this is certainly effective.

If we pay close attention, though, we sometimes see that it "feels good" or right to move towards and through, rather than dance around or past, our pain. As Neale Donald Walsch says in his *Conversations With God* book series, "What you look at disappears."[1] Pain does not generally persist if we do not feed it with further resistance, resentment, and fear. We do not have to run towards pain, but we don't want to run away from it. Our own presence is the truth that sets us free from pain.

Am I making light of pain? Perhaps, and sometimes this is a good thing. One of my teachers, a wonderful Sufi master named Jamal Rahman would often tell us, "Tremble with it." Compassionately being with and trembling with our pain is not suffering, but surrendering. When we shiver with our pain, we find that it does have an ending. Like a rain soaked dog, we shake ourselves free.

Still, when we are muddling in the middle of pain it is anything but easy. The healing process can be so mysterious, frustrating, and exhausting. Add to this the confusion as to how to heal, a less than supportive and sometimes unaffordable health care system, and perhaps many physical and emotional wounds coexisting simultaneously, we can easily become hopeless, depressed, or even suicidal.

Yet, we can remind ourselves of the deepest truth, that healing can be instantaneous, even miraculous. The limits we, or other well-meaning friends, healers, or doctors set may not be real in the truest sense. While we all experience pain at various points in our life--with the loss of a loved one, a life threatening disease, or less tragic bumps and bruises--we do have some choice over how we handle that pain. We do not have to feed our pain and turn it into suffering. We can ask: "What is this pain telling me?" Pain can be a teacher, a prod to presence. Stubbing your toe is a good lesson in slowing down. Heart problems may tell us we are pushing too hard, or not loving ourselves.

As I write this chapter, my back hurts, an ongoing challenge from a traumatic auto accident seven years ago. While the pain is still considerable, I do notice that when I fight it, it intensifies. When I judge myself, the other driver, my attorney, or the insurance company for the way the case was handled, I wallow in the past and suffer. When I project the situation into the future--*how will I make a living*?--the pain intensifies. But when I stay present, breathe deeply, practice compassion, and trust that things happen for a reason, that when one door closes (I had to quit a job, which I didn't particularly like) another opens (my health business has grown). Moreover, there may be an underlying and ongoing karmic balancing act that is always giving us exactly what we need.

With *emotional* pain, the hardest things for a "do something" culture is to just be with it, be patiently and attentively present, open to whatever arises. Let's say we are feeling jealousy. What color is it? What shape? Where is it residing in your body? Is it moving, or stagnant? Are there any secondary emotions that arise?

Breathe deeply and feel, listen, watch. There may be nothing to do, but be present, and see what happens, maybe a shift, maybe an insight, maybe nothing. It's all okay.

What *thoughts* might be feeding your physical or emotional pain? As the ego constantly strives for identity, we must be careful not to label ourselves as "wounded" or "diseased." We are not our pain, but rather infinite and everlasting Divine Beings.

Soul pain may be telling us we are not living our life to the fullest. Without pain to nudge us, we may never come to notice that we have abandoned our way. Again, we can be still and listen, provide space for that quieter voice to whisper its guidance--before it shouts and gets our attention in less gentle ways. Remember, this is our own voice, calling us to love. Do we have the courage to respond, take back our life, and find our passion? When we are fully alive and walking our path, there is less time for preoccupation with pain.

There is a crucial distinction here between self-indulgence in our pain from the mind or ego's perspective, and being fully present from the Being's perspective, giving it some necessary space, attention, and compassion. Ego attaches to and amplifies the suffering, while our Being decreases and dissipates the pain. Ego adds darkness and density, while Being evokes love and luminosity.

☙ Practice Points

- Be present whenever pain arises in your life. Is it physical, emotional, mental, or spiritual? Can you bring presence to the pain?

☙ Contemplation: Peace with Pain

- Tune in to any *physical* pain you are aware of: Just be with it, breathing deeply into it with compassionate awareness. Is the pain telling you anything? What does it need? Can you release any fear, resistance, or judgment of the pain?
- Tune in to any *emotional* pain or soul longing (this may be related to the physical pain). Again, just be with it, feel it, perhaps hear its message. Be present, fill your heart with compassion, and let your own transformative energy soften your pain.

ADDICTIONS

Habit is either the best of servants or the worst of masters.
- Nathaniel Emmons

We earlier looked at attachments, and addictions are simply very intense attachments. An addiction is sometimes described as an individual's continuing compulsion to engage in some particular activity, regardless of harmful consequences to that person's physical, mental, or emotional health, or overall life. Ending an addiction may include physical withdrawal symptoms and emotional angst. There may be many factors in addiction, including social, biological, and genetic.

What do you think or feel when you hear the word "addiction?" What images come to mind? Emotional or physical suffering? An addict in the street? Hopelessness? Shame? Guilt? Most likely a quite negative or even painful feeling, image, or memory is evoked.

Do you have any addictions? All of us have experienced pain, and all of us have done something to divert or deny the pain. When these diversions evolve into addictions, any dependency--whether gambling or web-surfing--causes suffering. We are wise to explore our attachments and compulsive activities.

As an example, let look at drugs--legal or illegal. Of course, prescription and other drugs are often helpful and necessary in our world. Psychiatric drugs may actually provide enough strength and stability to heal or begin the inner work. Furthermore, many native groups like the Huichol Indians in Mexico have used peyote for generations, in ritual to expand the mind. These uses of drugs are not necessarily unhealthy or even attachments. Yet most of us would benefit by striving to feel the fullness of life unaltered by tranquilizers and numbing agents, cleansing the temple and clearing our heads, to have any chance at an expansive life.

One hundred year old Miss West attributed her longevity to long walks, playing the piano, and taking the stairs instead of the elevator. But more important, she claims, "I don't take any medicine. I did once and got sick, so I knew enough to stop."[1]

America is now the most drugged nation on Earth. Five out of six Americans over age 65 are on at least one drug, and most are on several.[2] In the last chapter, we looked at ways to handle pain, but in the U.S., the use of painkillers nearly doubled between 1997 and 2005.[3] Now there are even polypills, which make it easier to take many pills in one capsule!

Government policies do not always support efforts to go clean, too often focusing on punishment and prisons, violent and costly drug wars abroad, with scarce investment in rehabilitation. We have a pharmaceutical industry with one of Washington D.C.'s most powerful and insidious lobbies. Dementia and Alzheimer's are tremendous problems in America, but some medical studies are finding that excessive prescription drugs may be causing some of the memory loss and delirium. There are now even medical terms to describe adverse health affects from the prescribing too many drugs or other excessive medical procedures to patients: "polypharmacy" and "iatrogenic illness."

One of my students had an ailing, elderly mother who was taking 13 pills a day, and eventually stopped eating, apparently preparing to die. The doctor told the family that they might as well stop the medications, as she was clearly in her last days. Free from the medications, her mother began eating, her health improved, and the last I heard she was doing well several months later. Many of these drugs simply mask the symptoms, prevent us from hearing the shouts of the body (and the Earth), and keep us from taking full responsibility for ourselves.

Some would argue that *any* habit is unhealthy. Even functional routines like a determined yoga or meditation practice can become obsessive, and we are wise to bring mindfulness to all our behaviors. Paradoxically, yoga can help us naturally overcome our addictions, vices, and compulsive behaviors, simply because we become more present.

Our addictions may have served us well for the short term. Cigarettes may have seemed like your only true friend, relieving a loneliness that felt like death to the soul. So, you found a friend that never puts you down, that never says no, a friend you can always count on. So, is quitting cold turkey always the loving thing to do?

The compassionate thing may be to begin a friendship with *yourself*, practice trusting yourself and then others a bit more. We come to see that cigarettes are a poor substitute for genuine connection and community.

Like food issues, addictions tie into lower chakra survival instincts. The body believes it needs the addiction to survive. So, loving ourselves means communicating with the body, practicing kindness, going slowly, and eventually learning to replace the addiction with true needs.

What we really need, as with any form of pain or suffering, is our own company, the healing vibration of our essential Self showing up, comforting the body, recognizing the patterns, and choosing something more liberating and life giving. Eventually, the compulsive and life-draining aspects of the addiction will be replaced by precious presence, trust, and unrestricted freedom.

෨ Practice Points

- Be the silent and compassionate witness to yourself.
- When you feel compelled or compulsive, take a couple deep breaths to evoke presence. Ask yourself: What am I feeling? What do I *really* need? How can I love myself more in this situation?

෨ Contemplation

- As a child, did members of your family have addictions? What kinds? What did this teach you?
- Look at an attachment or addiction you have. Release any judgment you may have about it. What need is this filling? Can you thank it?
- What are you really seeking? Can you learn to give this to yourself? Release any belief that you cannot have what you really need.
- Breath of compassion. Sense your profound power; and know that with love and support you can overcome anything.

DEPRESSION AND GRIEF

Research suggests that unexpressed feelings locked in the body form focal points of tension and stress that may eventually contribute to the development of life-threatening illnesses such as cancer and heart disease.
 - Stephan Bodian

Depression is the repression of expression. We repress, or press down, our very self, our life, our sexuality, our personality, and our Divinity. We deny our painful feelings: sadness, grief, or anger. When we do this, we also lock away our life force: our joy, silliness, laughter. We thus bury our very reason for being here: our passion, purpose, and gifts. No wonder we are depressed!

Signs of depression include anxiety, loneliness, fatigue, hopelessness, helplessness, inability to feel pleasure, and insomnia. How serious is this? Nearly 20 million Americans suffer from depression in any given year. We just mentioned our attachment to drugs; well, doctors wrote 190 million prescriptions for antidepressants in the U.S. in 2006.[1] One out of every ten Americans is now taking antidepressants--double the amount in 1996.[2] England also mirrored our antidepressant increase. Interestingly, many of the studies suggest that placebos work about as well as antidepressant drugs, without the often considerable side effects.

There are also about 30,000 suicides in the U.S. each year, or an average of 85 each day. Some recent studies argue that Americans are some of the least happy and most depressed people in the world.[3]

Why are we so depressed anyway? In one sense, if you are not depressed, you are not paying attention, as the mess we have made here on Earth can be depressing! Like hamsters innocently but frantically running in place, we have good intentions, but simply do not know how to unwind ourselves from the rat (or hamster) race.

Stress levels seem to match the rise in our technological dependence. In one study in 2006, eighty-five percent of consumers say they've sworn, shouted, cried, smashed things, or experienced chest pains while waiting for help on tech-support call lines.[4] So, even when we do allow ourselves to express emotions, it is often more of an explosion than a healthy release.

Other ways of describing depression are compressed, constricted, or disconnected from the Divine. One dictionary definition of depression is *dispirited*. Could it be this simple? Have we lost our Spirit, our essential link and lifeline to what nourishes the soul? A *Course in Miracles* teaches, "When you equate yourself with a body you will always experience depression."[5]

We heal when we come fully into the body, honor the messages of the body, and integrate everything that lives there. And every energy--especially depression--needs the vitality of motion, so the hamster wheel has its place. It is hard to be depressed when you are active, doing something you enjoy. Exercise or sports, or other movement, such as yoga, tai chi, or swimming help elevate the pleasure neurotransmitter dopamine (although sometimes *over*-activity like the internet, video games, and drugs can *deplete* the dopamine). There is no simple one-size-fits-all solution; you find what works for you.

Sometimes the roots of depression are more physiological than emotional, so environmental or nutritional changes can be very helpful. Cutting back on sugars or caffeine may help. Omega-3 fatty acids, such as fish oil, and Vitamin B Complex can be important. Eat regularly to maintain the energy and the blood sugar level. In addition, testing for allergies such as wheat can be critical.

Here in the Pacific Northwest, many people get the winter blues from the cloudy winter grays. Often people say, "I just wish it would rain; I hate this overcast." This is like stifled tears. When the crying-clouds finally release and the tears flow, we feel a cleansing and cathartic release, and liberation from pain. Most of us have an accumulation of unshed tears--let them flow. Know that every tear is helping wash the sting of past wounds from the body, and life grows where water falls.

Grief is somewhat different from depression--although repressed grief can turn to depression. It is human, natural, and even healthful to feel and acknowledge sadness and grief, which is simply the release of sorrow around a loss, whether it is a grandmother or a baseball game. There is a time to feel the breaking of bonds from someone we were energetically connected to. Or, it may be the moment to let go of a certain stage in your life, a career, or to honor the sadness of an empty nest. The grief has an ending, unless you suspend the feelings and allow it to distort into bitterness or hopelessness.

It is important to honor your own timetable concerning grief; no one can tell you how to do it or how long to grieve. Take special care of your body during this time, and try not to cut corners or numb yourself with drugs or alcohol. Other emotions may naturally arise during the grieving process: anger, confusion, fear. Breathe deeply. It may help to ask for help, to cry, or be alone. Give it space to run its course, but by all means grieve your losses. William Cowper said, "Grief itself is a medicine."[6]

As we learn this art of being human, we allow ourselves to inhabit the body and feel fully, knowing that this too passes, that this too is part of the path and the gift of being human. Time will take away cars, homes, and even loved ones, to which we can healthfully grieve, and give gratitude for the time we had together.

Depression is an opportunity to move from half aliveness to full living. When you feel as if you are going mad, it may in fact be your Soul shaking you free from your ego identification. It can be the end of "business as usual" and the start of living in line with your deepest values, your soul calling, and purpose. Can we let go of the old and open to the new? Joy and liberation await us.

We once endured a Great Depression, and now we are living the Great Expression. The earth energy shifts are highlighting any lies and illusions, and we are being shaken awake and free. We are moving from the survival of the ruthless to the thriving of an evolving Earth and those who turn to the new-old way of community, sustainability, and love.

ᏚᎤ Practice Points:
5 Tips for Handling Depression and Grief

1. Feel fully. Don't be in a hurry to get "rid" of the grief or depression.
2. Paradoxically, don't let your depression depress you! Give it some space, but don't get stuck there. Move your body. Try yoga, nature walks, or sports.

3. Community. Depression invites--and can be deepened by--isolation. Try connecting with friends, asking for help, or visiting a support group or therapist.
4. See a naturopath. Get a checkup to rule out allergies and nutritional deficiencies.
5. Passion. Do what you enjoy; make time for fun.

✑ Contemplation: Compassionate Presence

- Breathe slowly and deeply for a couple of minutes to invite presence.
- Bring attention to the heart, and fill it with compassion.
- Invite any feelings of sadness, loss, or grief to arise, and bring them to the comfort of your heart.
- Take a deep breath and say hello to the feeling. Let it be. Let it talk to you. Listen, like a good friend. If tears come, let them flow freely.

NEVER GIVE UP

Until you've kept your eyes and your wanting still for fifty years, you don't begin to cross over from confusion.
- Rumi

Ever wonder where a river starts? What begins as a drip joins with other drops and flows into a trickle, then gathers runoff and momentum from snowfields, creeks or streams, and evolves into a raging river, emptying into lakes or back into the ocean itself.

Most of us have seen "waves" at sporting events, where the crowd raises its arms, stands, and creates a flowing human wave around the stadium. Once, at a Seattle Mariner baseball game, I witnessed the birth of a wave. A young man got our attention by facing up towards the crowd, shouting, pointing the direction the wave was to flow, then counted down: 3 . . . 2 . . . 1 . . . Whooo! We jumped to our feet, shouted, raised our arms, and then watched as the human wave started strong but fizzled out over the next couple of sections. After a dozen attempts, this young man with a now-gravelly voice was undaunted. He gathered some young helpers, and reversed the direction of the wave. Soon, I was more entertained by this man's persistent efforts than the game itself. Eventually, he encouraged the wave to spread ever further, until tens of thousands of people carried the wave around the entire stadium.

Personal and global transformation take courageous commitment, and we must never give up. Whether we are starting a wave, beating a cancer, or stopping a war, we are so capable--especially when we work together. It may not be the quick fix so popularly advertised, but with perseverance, we *will* be transformed, for wholeness is our nature.

Perhaps there can be a smart stubbornness and a stupid stubbornness. There is a place for giving up, a healthy aspect of surrender that we explored earlier. This is where we stop our compulsive and egotistical need to push and control things, blindly and bullishly.

There is also a very unhealthy side to surrender, where we give up hope, assume that the cause is lost, that the Earth and our political system or our personal challenges are beyond resuscitation. If we believe there is no chance for change, we create exactly that reality in our life and world. We can be quite dramatic; we can give up and throw our hands in the air--not in a wave, but to pronounce the world evil--or maybe just unfixable.

When I began studying and receiving hands-on energy healing work, at times I felt hopeless, completely lost in the surfacing pain and suffocating anxiety. One gifted and sensitive healer, Jackie, who worked on me, told me years later that when she first put her hands on me she almost fainted from all the fear and pain she could feel in my body. At times, I felt that life was not worth the struggle, but I am so glad I did not quit.

My friend Cheri O'Brien never gave up. Rather than shut down when she developed breast cancer, she blossomed, took trips and vacations and had fun. She not only defeated the cancer, but continued and expanded her creative artwork, and is now one of the most successful artists I know.

Winston Churchill said, "Success is going from failure to failure without loss of enthusiasm."[1] In the United States, individuals and groups continue to organize, educate, and speak out for progressive change. Despite a concentrated, corporate influence over much of our media and entertainment, people are using the internet, blogs, public television, and other media to express and share progressive perspectives and invite conscious dialogue. We have millions of what are now called "Cultural Creatives,"--conscious and compassionate healers who think outside the box and are creating new paradigms. Then we have the "Indigo children"--gifted or advanced souls who are showing up to assist our world at this time of transition.

On the way home from that baseball game, I noticed plants squeezing out from between the cracks in the concrete highway barriers. The drive to live and grow is unstoppable. Human beings have an indomitable spirit, and the search for truth and the desire to help one another are all natural expressions of who we are at the deepest level. Evil, fear, poverty, and war all have an ending, but love does not.

The daily news may reveal chaos. Yet, for every pain, there is unimaginable heroism. For every act of violence, there are countless reports of compassion and service. For every nation at war, ten more are at peace. Some studies show that wars are actually on the decline in our world. In 2005, an exhaustive report by researchers at the University of British Columbia found that since 1991, despite the violence in Rwanda, Iraq, Afghanistan, and the Balkans, the number of conflicts actually fell by at least 40 percent. The number of deaths per war dropped by a whopping 98 percent from an average of 38,000 to 600 by 2002.[2]

In our quest for truth, healing, and wholeness--whatever we seek--we need never give up on our task. As Gandhi and Martin Luther King, Jr. said, the glory is in the struggle, not the results. We can release attachment to outcome and get to work.

In the end, there actually is no struggle. Know that at the deepest level, North and South, rich and poor, Christian and Muslim, rightwing and leftwing, blue state and red state, gay and straight, black and white—we are all One. Regardless of whatever has caused us to forget, with patience and perseverance, we shall surely overcome.

"Never give up, no matter what is going on. Never give up. Develop the heart. Too much energy in your country is spent developing the mind instead of the heart. Develop the heart. Be compassionate... Never give up!"[3]
- The Dalai Lama

ᖬ Practice Points

- Notice those moments when you feel like quitting. See if you can notice the difference between smart stubbornness and silly stubbornness.

ᖬ Contemplation: Never Give Up.

- Take a deep breath, and connect with your deepest Self. Feel the fullness, the power, the joy.
- Validate your courage and resilience. Reflect on some specific past example or evidence of your staying power, a time when you refused to give up, regardless of the outcome. How did that feel?

OWN YOUR DARK SIDE

The only devils in the world are those running around in our hearts. That is where the battle should be fought.
- Gandhi

We may say that the devil made us do it, but our human personalities all have a touch of d-evil in us. Evil is simply pain and hate vented or expressed outwards, and it has a range or degree of meanness. It may be expressed by dropping a wise comment or setting off a bomb.

Devil spelled backwards is *lived*, and anyone who has lived in a human body has a shadow that needs the light of love. Aleksandr Solzhenitsyn said, "If only it were all so simple! If only there were evil people somewhere insidiously committing evil deeds, and it were necessary only to separate them from the rest of us and destroy them. But the line dividing good and evil cuts through the heart of every human being."[1]

There is a story of a woman looking for her keys under a streetlight. A man comes by and offers to help, asking, "Where did you last see the keys?" "Over in that dark forest," she replies. Puzzled, the man asks, "Then why are you looking *here*?" To which she replies, "Here, there is more light."

Few of us, understandably, want to look too closely into the dark, or gaze into our scary shadows. There is a workshop I conduct called *Dancing in the Dark: Healing our Shadows*. It is about as popular as my *Healing the Feelings* workshop; few people ever show up.

A Course in Miracles says, "The escape from darkness involves two stages: First, the recognition that darkness cannot hide. This step usually entails fear. Second, the recognition that there is nothing you want to hide, even if you could. This step brings escape from fear. When you have become willing to hide nothing, you will not only be willing to enter into communion but will also understand peace and joy."[2]

Darkness and light are part of our human dichotomy and drama. Our truest Selves may be light and bright, but our human selves have some muck and mold. Again, these unconscious emotions and traits are not necessarily *bad*; they are simply and naturally part of our developing human experience, until they are not.

I have had numerous students who come for meditation class tell me that their motivation is to release stress and find their center. I applaud their courage, for valor is required to meditate. I also mention that sometimes it gets more uncomfortable before it gets better. When we finally sit still in meditation, some shadowy aspects may emerge, and this is good! Most of us have spent a lifetime avoiding looking too closely at our fury, our fear, our indignity, so we keep them in the shadows. Some students simply do not come back, "I came here to feel good, not worse."

Some perspective may help, for this is not an easy time to be embodied on Earth. According to many Hindu scholars, we are currently nearing the end of the Kali Yuga, an Earth age that is sometimes known as the "Dark Age." It is believed to be a challenging era of spiritual degeneration and disconnect from God--but is only one of four cycles or eras. We are already entering the next stage, or "yuga," which promises to be much more bright.

It has been said that if a man loves God, he will heal and become holy in ten years. But if she hates God, she can do the same in one year. If hate is within us, it needs movement. When we side-step the shadows and deny the darkness, we only delay the dawn. Again, we all eventually hit our dark night of the soul. Some of us may move through it in a weekend, while others take a thousand lifetimes--there is no hurry. Some of us have less dramatic incarnations with no discernable battles, while others have epic struggles.

This is the classic battle we see in the *Bhagavad Gita*. In a conversation between Arjuna (the seeker) and Krishna (the Divine Presence), Arjuna struggles with the decision of going to war or not. Shall he annihilate his dark side? Would this not diminish him, by destroying a part of himself? Krishna seems to argue that these dark energies are not actually a part of his truest Self, and so he must eradicate them.

But is this true? And if so, how do we eradicate them? It is open to interpretation. Love is the greatest healer: does it destroy or transform? Or both? When we bring the higher energy vibration of our own loving presence, we begin the process of highlighting and healing, unearthing the raw gems within the buried energies. Each contraction that we face, embrace, and breathe into softens, and releases stuck or stored life force energy, and we feel lighter, enlivened.

Hate, shame, anger--they all live in the darkness of your unexplored mind. They transform and integrate with love, light, and open air. Whatever is there, pop the lid and look directly at it, feel it, breathe into it. Discuss it with your partner, therapist, or friend. Roll around in the muck!

The Tao te Ching says, "Darkness within darkness. The gateway to all understanding."[3] Within the layer of *stuff* is the glory and the gold, which we will miss if we quit the inner work prematurely. If we stop digging, or if we lack focus or commitment and dig countless shallow holes in too many directions, we will only delay the treasure.

It takes boldness to bring a nonjudgmental presence to our

wimpy and warty sides. Martin Luther King, Jr. said, "Darkness cannot drive out darkness; only light can do that. Hate cannot drive out hate; only love can do that."[4] We may be blinded when we see our essential brightness, and maybe this, our true and unrestricted light, frightens us more than any dark.

℘ Practice Points

- Notice when you feel vengeful, jealous, nasty, or hateful. Can you bring presence, acceptance, and acknowledgement to these shadowy elements of your personality?

℘ Contemplation: Entering the Shadow

- Breathe deeply and assure your body that you are safe.
- Imagine approaching a dark cave, where some lost aspects of yourself live. Stay grounded and connected with your breath, and inquire within. What lies in your shadows? What part of you is asking for the light of your conscious presence? Greet with compassion whatever shadow-self you meet. Listen more, speak less. Thank it for the visit, and promise to return and listen again sometime.

PART SIX: POWER, PURPOSE, AND PASSION

OWN YOUR LIGHT SIDE

Only full, overhead sun diminishes your shadow.
- Rumi

We just peeked into the shadows, and earlier we looked at those who mirror our raw, unpolished, or painful areas. We now invite acknowledgment of our positive traits, reflected by those we admire, our heroes whose qualities we may also possess. We don't visit the shadows to stay sulking in darkness. As with a buried seed, we can emerge like sunflowers, facing towards and standing tall in the sunlight.

One would think that we are more afraid of our deep dark shadows than our bigness and brightness, but this is not necessarily true. We both desire and dread our light. In our workshops, it is always easier for people to recognize their own negative aspects mirrored back by other people, rather than the positive reflection of their own golden gifts, talents, and greatness.

As mentioned earlier under the "Feeling Feelings" chapter, we generally inhabit a middle zone of familiarity throughout most of our lives, where we tend to avoid both the dark and the light, our shadows as well as our shining. Examine it in your own life. Do you avoid both the pain as well as true pleasure? Are you mired in the midst of mediocrity?

When stuck in my deepest muck in my early forties, I was often terrified, ashamed, or fuming. When people laughed or joked around, it rattled and irritated me. It felt like the higher frequency of energy associated with laughter and joy smacked squarely against my painful, denser energy body, jarring me and triggering fury at whoever was disturbing my misery!

We often choose the illusion of safety and familiarity over the adventure of unfamiliar territory or the risk of exposure. The solution may be to gradually expand the range of your comfort zone of feelings and experience. You can greet the sharks of the shadows--which really have no teeth--welcoming their lessons and gifts, and transforming the energies back into life. These energies free and feed the love that already lives within you, so you literally raise your energy vibration, and allow more joy, light, and passion in your life. It's a beautiful cycle; the more light you bring in, the brighter you shine.

Here we are not referring to the enjoyment of sipping a beer after work, watching the latest popular movie, or buying a fashionable outfit. The worldly pleasures we seek are poor substitutes for the genuine aliveness we may feel when speaking our truth or pursuing our true mission. We often find time for everything except that which really matters, and we limit our pleasure to mundane and shallow external entertainment--if any at all. But we have a life awaiting us!

When we stand bright, we get some attention, and we may love this as well as fear this. People will begin to rely on us, give us more responsibility, or urge us into leadership roles. Bright lights may attract allies, but also moths! When we stand tall, or stand out, people notice and some may try to knock us back down. They certainly shot Jesus down, as they later did Mahatma Gandhi, Martin Luther King, Jr., and countless others who knew that their Soul mission overrode the human risk.

But along with the moths, these heroes also attracted and invited the best in people. Jesus lit up the world with his light and love; no cave or tomb could hold him in the dark. Some of us focus on the dark side of Jesus' life--his death and suffering--but his bigger message was one of eternal light and life.

We are wise to watch the company we keep, as we tend to match the energy vibration of those around us. In the word guru, *gu* means darkness, and *ru* means light. A guru is one who can help hold the energy, light up our shadows until we ourselves can step forth from the dark and maintain the charge. When we acknowledge and honor the light in the guru or another, we actually brighten ourselves. Then we can help light up the world.

We all have the same sacred roots. You are gifted, magnificent, and exceptional, just like everyone else. We all have the potential to shine with the same intensity, when we allow our distinctive luminosity.

Practice Points

- Be attentive to how you feel when you meet people who are successful, bright, or powerful. Is there envy or support? Jealousy or appreciation? These can be clues to how much of your own greatness you allow.
- Practice maintaining your brightness, even when others feel or act diminished or competitive.

Contemplation: Golden Mirrors

- Breathe deeply. Similar to what we did in the "Relationships as Mirrors" section earlier, reflect on three people you admire or see as heroes. What are the main traits you admire about them?
- Ask yourself: Do I have these traits--perhaps undeveloped? Have I ever allowed, or could I ever demonstrate, these traits?

ILLUMINATING THE ILLUSIONS

The knowledge that illuminates not only sets you free, but also shows you clearly that you already are free.
- A Course in Miracles

Webster's defines *illuminate* as "to give light to; to light up; to make clear." The very next entry down the page, we find the word *illusion*, defined as "a false idea or conception; an unreal or misleading image or appearance."[1]

My goal in writing this book is to help add to the light that is increasingly highlighting the dark in our world. While it is important to accept and learn from our pain and suffering, what can we do to stop creating so darned much of it!? How can we change our personal and global energy and environment to help illuminate the illusions, and therefore eradicate our suffering?

The 14th Dalai Lama said, "In Buddhism, ignorance as the root cause of suffering refers to a fundamental misperception of the true nature of the self and all phenomena."[2] As with the yoga perspective, the Buddha taught that misperception causes much pain in our world, and that we all suffer. Both Patanjali and the Buddha believed we could curtail future anguish by following certain steps.

The Noble Eightfold Path, as taught by Siddhartha Gautama, the Buddha, describes the path to end suffering: right view, right intention, right speech, right action, right livelihood, right effort, right mindfulness, and right concentration.

The "right" in this sense is not a judgment as in good or bad, but rather that which serves us, helps us awaken, and stops creating future suffering. It is a practical guideline to mental development, aimed at freeing us from attachments and delusions. The ultimate goal is realizing the truth in all things. The Eightfold Path makes up the heart of Buddhism, together with the Four Noble Truths:

1. Suffering is part of life.
2. Attachment and grasping cause suffering.
3. We can end suffering.
4. The Eightfold Path can liberate us from suffering.

The Eightfold Path has some overlap with the Eight Limbs of Yoga, which include: *yamas* (behavior in the world, such as nonviolence and honesty), *niyamas* (personal codes of conduct, such as nutrition, self study, and prayer), *asana* (yoga poses), *pranayama* (breath regulation), *pratyahara* (withdrawal of the senses--coming home to the body), *dharana* (concentration), *dhyana* (meditation, or absorption), and *samadhi* (bliss or super consciousness). Both Buddhists and Yogis teach that we can dispel suffering by illuminating our illusions.

Again and again, we practice *attention* and *intention*. We decide that if there is something we are ignoring, that if all of us humans have limited vision so to speak, we hold an intention of waking up. With practice, we open our mind, eye, and heart to the truth of who we are and what we are here to do. We listen, for the universe will show us how. Rumi said, "There is a way between voice and presence where information flows. In disciplined silence, it opens. With wandering talk it closes."[3]

As you seek a path through the world of delusion, you can start to notice: do Buddhist principles help? Does yoga work? Attending Unity, Interfaith, or other churches? Does Christianity touch my soul? Islam? No-ism? What awakens, stirs me to deeper meaning, so that the confusion is no longer overwhelming, but just a passing wave, like the many thoughts that cross the mind?

Our Presence illuminates. There is no darkness that our own conscious awareness cannot brighten and lighten. When light encounters darkness, light wins. Imagine being inside the biggest indoor stadium; if you light one tiny match, all that darkness cannot extinguish it.

This is not an all-or-nothing experience or concept. We all have dimmer switches, most of which are turned way down due to worries and wounds. But our collective dimmer switch is rising, making it easier and safer for each of us to risk raising our personal energy level. As we grow accustomed to ever more light, the shift from ignorance and illusion to magnificence and illumination accelerates. On Earth at this very moment, we are moving into a wonderful era where what is hidden becomes visible, and what needs healing will become apparent.

We *eliminate* our ignorance and suffering by *illuminating* it. We shine the light of our awareness, the brilliance of our own conscious presence, onto and into all areas of ourselves and our lives. We come to see the changing nature of this material world, and remember the deepest, Divine Reality that surrounds and penetrates it, that which we are.

By persistent and sustained practice, anyone and everyone can make the yoga journey and reach the goal of illumination and freedom. Krishna, Buddha, and Jesus lie in the hearts of all.[4]

- B.K.S. Iyengar

∞ Practice Points

- Practice slowing down and being more present: Allow the light of your conscious presence into your daily activities.

∞ Contemplation

- Take a few deep breaths, noticing the four parts of breath: in breath, pause, out breath, pause.
- Imagine an open flow of clear communication and light down through the energy center at the top of your head (crown chakra). Feel the whole body brighten and lighten. Ask the universe to guide you to whatever you need to know.

COMMITMENT TO YOUR PATH

Concerning all acts of initiative and creation, there is one elementary truth-- that the moment one definitely commits oneself, then Providence moves, too.
- Johann Wolfgang Von Goethe

What is your path? The key word here is *your*. There are many paths, crossroads, and choices in life. Only you--you and your deepest truth--can choose the path that is best for you. But is there only one right path or are there several? Are we punished or do we suffer if we choose the wrong path? How much time and energy have you spent searching for--or fearfully avoiding--your path?

You may not know who you are. You may have given your power away so much that you have forgotten that your needs count. You may be so disconnected from your feelings that you have no idea what brings you joy. Our perfectionist and fearful minds have us dreading failure or the "wrong" decision and the inevitable consequences of our mistakes. So, we settle or freeze.

What made us so afraid? Where is our passion? We have a free country, yet our minds and egos are often in control, and therefore we are anything but free. Furthermore, like drinking alcohol, our minds are *under the influence* of our external environment, the cacophony of family or cultural voices, and our societal "norms." *Normal* is not always healthy or healing! Normal is being led by outside authority figures that are often lost themselves. We are told we should get an education, we should go to college, we should get a PhD., we should be a doctor or an attorney. Or, perhaps we shouldn't go to college--that's for rich or smart people. We should be a waiter, or take over the family business, get to work and make money now. Either way, we choose from fear.

Ralph Waldo Emerson said, "Do not follow where the path may lead. Go instead where there is no path and leave a trail."[1] Regardless of what the "experts" say, (*including the Bible, Yoga Sutras, Bhagavad Gita, Koran,* or *Torah)*, we can re-establish trust, connection, and confidence with our own truth. If people, gurus, books, or writings touch your heart and highlight your path, use them, but stay connected with your Self.

When we align with the Divine, our human will is not separate from the higher will. When we are connected to our breath, when we have cleared the emotional excesses, we come to trust the inner voice as the same with the One Voice. Our world needs all of us to stop doubting our deepest Selves and know that where there is a passion, there is a path. With a heartfelt trust, we can walk through the haze of uncertainty, knowing that our next step will become visible. The old ways begin to naturally close down behind us and propel us forward.

In both Yoga and in Buddhism--or any quality teaching or religion--we are not given answers but asked questions. We are invited into our own experience, and offered tools that may help us find our own path. It is said, "If you follow the herd, you'll step in a lot of poop." When we follow others, the view always remains the same, and it ain't pretty. The closer we follow, the more it stinks!

A few years back, I was desperately praying for guidance for my path, believing I would never find it or accomplish anything, and judging the heck out of myself. I sent my first book in to an editor, who deflated my writing ambitions, telling me quite directly that I was hardly an authority figure that people would take seriously. But, I had a passion to write, and God plays no tricks.

I finally made a commitment to self publish, and felt a shift of energy, like a refreshing summer breeze. I knew that in seeking approval of a potential publisher--who supposedly knew more than me--I had been writing someone else's book. Suddenly, I was writing *my* book, from the heart rather than fear. The other book was gone and this book took its place. If we have a will, we have a way.

There is not some judgmental and castigating bearded dude in the sky waiting to punish us for not following the "right" path. It is true, though, that the path we choose has consequences, and if we do not follow our own *dharma* (path or duty), we may feel incompletion, resentment, or depression. When one person withholds their gifts or a part of themselves, it is a loss for all of us. Henry Van Dyke said, "Use what talents you possess. The woods would be very silent if no birds sang there except those that sang best."[2]

When you make a choice of path, remember that it may be for a day, or a lifetime. So do not become attached to friends, mates, money, jobs, or paths--nothing. Focus and commit, yes, but moment to moment, we must be flexible and attentive and trust what feels right.

Not knowing your path is a good place to start. Sometimes not knowing keeps us from entering too soon, keeps us focused on something else first, which itself is part of the path. If fear, doubt, and confusion have held you back, then fear, doubt, and confusion are presently part of your path. If you are not feeling a sense of joy and fulfillment in your life, then be with the path of emptiness or lack. Everything is our path, for it is beneath our feet, here and now. This is the essence of Zen.

What gives you joy? What touches your heart? The benevolent and abundant universe often offers us clues. For example, my last name is Holman, as in *whole human*. After years of disembodied living, I am learning, practicing, and now teaching others how to be fully in the body.

Another clue to your path: What once gave you great joy may also have gotten you in trouble. You may have been invalidated for your zeal, by limiting, jealous, or wounded people. You may be a good listener, cook, organizer, dancer, writer, leader, mathematician, waitperson, or body worker. Trust yourself and make your passion your path. Whatever invites a song in your heart or a silly smile on your face is a sacred gift to our world.

When you do find something, enter it with as much passion

and commitment as you can muster. Clear the mind of as much of the doubt, chatter, and critical voices as possible, and jump in with guts and gusto. This is the land of magic and miracles, where the mysterious forces of the universe back you easily, naturally, magnificently.

My mother loved to sing, but her life choices and low self-esteem restrained her voice. She sometimes told us that she wished she could return in her next life as a singer, and her last words before she died were, "Let's all sing a song." May we not wait too long to sing our song.

෨ Practice Points

- During your daily activities, notice which ones help you feel alive and which ones drain you.
- Notice when daydreams arise--what are they saying?

෨ Contemplation: Your Path

- Breathe, and reflect: What would you like to commit to and make priorities for in your life?
- What is your mission? If you have no clue, ask the universe or God. Trust that you will be guided, and be open to how this guidance presents itself.

POWER UP!

It is our duty--as men and women--to behave as though limits to our own ability do not exist. We are co-creators of the Universe.
- Pierre Teilhard de Chardin

I once went to a refreshing Catholic service where the priest, a fiery man named Jack Morris said, "The church is primarily about the people of God. We are all of equal importance, and we all need to be consulted and called into the dialogue. The laity are not uneducated peasants whose sole tasks are to pay, pray and obey."

Jack was right; in a new world, we will have less control, hierarchy, and power *over* others (over powering), and more genuine empowerment and active participation by we the people. Growing up in a quite authoritarian and abusive Catholic school system, I quickly absorbed the message that others knew more than me. Hell, they seemed to have a direct line to heaven--or hell. It took many painful years before I could begin to recognize, appreciate, and allow my own voice and personal power.

Our healthy power and brightness are so necessary in this fearful, stressful world, a world in which many of us have been taught that power is bad and destructive. True, we often see power abused, and it is said that power itself corrupts. Frances Moore Lappé, in her book *Getting a Grip*, writes about redefining the word power. She writes of a teacher friend who asked his tenth graders what comes to mind when they hear the word *power*, and they responded "money, parents, guns, bullies, and Adolf Hitler."[1] Many of us have seen what power is, and we want none of it. Conversely, we want all of it, so that others will not hurt, bully, or control us.

Nevertheless, we hurt others and ourselves by hiding or denying our authentic power. Rather than power over other people and the Earth itself, we seek a power over ourselves. We gain the upper Mind over our little mind. We find power over our hurtful thoughts, egos, judgments, worries, and worldly temptations.

Nothing squelches our power like denial--whether it is of our feelings, body wisdom, or our unlimited power potential itself. So many of us have constricted the life out of ourselves; it will take some time to free our energies, but unleashed power is liberating. Recall that wonderful scene from the movie, *Network*, where people finally release their fear and begin shouting from their windows, "I'm mad as hell, and I'm not going to take it anymore!"

Too often, we have allowed madness to run our world, perhaps ironically, because we do not want to be as crazed or loud as the madmen who run things. But the madmen are deeply afraid of our true power. The meek *will* inherit the Earth, since meek does not mean weak; it simply means those who do not violate others.

When parents or teachers are ill at ease with their own power, they cannot be comfortable when little Johnny or Samantha begins to demonstrate his or her own (third chakra) exercises in will. More often than not, they will slam the door on even the healthy exhibits and experiments in self-assertion. We even call the youngest assertions of power the "terrible twos." The child learns to succumb to the "real" world of victims and helplessness.

We can surrender ego power to pure power. Again, this does not have to be unrealistic (there are few five foot basketball players in the NBA, although you never know), but simply holding true to the truth of who we are and our true potential. Jesus was not lying when he said, "... and greater works than these shall he do ..."[2] We can fly or walk on water, as long we are clearly inspired from our Soul and not our ego--in which case we will go splat or splash.

My friend Bev was once agonizing over a decision whether to leave the college where she had been teaching yoga for many years, to take another good job teaching gardening and nutrition. After weeks of worry, she finally came up with an idea she hadn't even considered: ask if she could alter the hours of the new job and keep *both* jobs. She was shocked and delighted when they easily agreed with her ideal situation. She recognized her power to create what she really wanted.

When we hold false limits and restricting images in our mind's eye, then that is what we will see manifest in our personal and collective life. If we believe that we must all compete with one another, work forty or sixty hours each week, and beg and borrow to survive and pay the bills, then so it is. But we can do so much better! Ralph Waldo Emerson said, "We are very near to greatness: one step and we are safe; can we not take the leap?"[3]

When we doubt or fear our power, we simply give power to the doubt and fear. What if we were to trust that there truly are no limits except for those created in our frail little minds and egos? As Arthur C. Clarke says, "The only way to discover the limits of the possible is to go beyond them into the impossible."[4]

⊗ Practice Points

- Notice thoughts or words that demonstrate limits, powerlessness, or negativity.
- Practice shifting to an open attitude and empowered words and action, and stay open to unbounded possibilities.

∞ Contemplation: Validate your Power.

- Breathe deeply and connect with your deepest Self. Reflect on how powerful you truly are--feel your power.
- Recall moments or situations when you demonstrated your healthy power. How did this feel? Scary? Good? Scary *and* good?

WAKE UP!

In the garden of gentle sanity may you be bombarded by coconuts of wakefulness.
- Chögyam Trungapa Rinpoche

Have you ever asked the front desk of a hotel to give you a wakeup call? Similarly, consciously or not, we may ask our teachers, spiritual guides, or deepest Self to give us a nudge when we have fallen into the illusion. Do we hear our own call? Do we ignore the prod, or the words of a song that touch your heart? Or do we ignore the heart attack? We can awaken to the message of each and every moment.

I recall a time I was put on hold, stuck in the branches of an automated phone tree. As I began to mope and sigh, aware of all the time I was "wasting," a recorded song came over the phone, with lyrics that went something like this: *Wake up wake up, to the sounds all around you...Can you feel the love...?* How's that for a wakeup call? Perhaps we can even turn phone tree hell into a heavenly moment.

Awakening is a fundamental swing in the way we see and experience the world and ourselves. It isn't necessarily something we can create, plan, or prepare for. Grace is often the seed to awakening. For reasons we may never understand, we are blessed with precious moments of aliveness, clarity, love, or otherworldly understanding. Do not hurry past these moments. In yoga they call this samadhi, when the veils of illusion part and we get a glimpse behind the curtain, beyond the superficial land of materialism and separation to the deeper world of spiritual Oneness.

The ideas we are exploring in this book--meditation, stillness, yoga, healthy relationships, sacred space--may help set the table for this most welcome guest of grace and its gift of awakening. We learn to pay attention so we do not miss the magic in every moment. We express our intention to be awakened from our sleep, and we may like what we open our eyes to. Persevering with our practice helps us return to that which we are, have been, and always will be. We can make grace our moment-to-moment reality.

When we awaken, we experience all that for which we have sought and struggled, only to see that it was always here. Until we are ready, it seems that no one tells us that what we are looking for is ourselves. In the nation of Bhutan, rather than a GNP (Gross National Product) to calculate and emphasize purely economic success, they use GNH (Gross National Happiness). The GNH index is an attempt to define quality of life in more holistic or even spiritual terms than GNP. Value is placed on wholeness and contentment, and this may stir an even greater awakening.

This book is about changing the Earth from the inside out. When we awaken spiritually, we reform socially, politically, and economically. Inner healing is a subversive act. When we learn to breathe, be present, and gain a clear attunement with our feelings and intuitions, we are powerful and global citizens who are not easily fooled or manipulated.

As we do our inner work, though, we can simultaneously make changes in the "outer" layers, or socioeconomic and political arenas. It is hard to meditate or awaken when we or our children are hungry, or exposed to environmental toxins. In the United States, there are numerous necessary reforms which would free up our minds and hearts, including: committing to a green and sustainable economy, campaign finance reform, progressive tax restructuring, healthcare reform that focuses on health rather than profits, and an education system that teaches essentials--emotional literacy, nonviolent communication, natural health, nutrition, earth care, and so on. True democratic policies and ideals--such as the Social Security and National Parks systems we enjoy--reawaken the soul of America.

What better time to awaken than now? Our world needs us each to show up, stand up, and to stop pretending that there are no problems. We can face the fact that ego has led us into dangerous territory, and take our power back over the madness of the most dangerous of leaders: our own unexplored mind.

There are beings that live much of their lives in an awakened state, and perhaps you know one of these people. They stand out, not necessarily because they do something grand or spectacular--although some of them do--but often since they are simply present, kind, in touch with their joy and heart. Their eyes dance with life, their words echo truth, and their lives are filled with passion. The Dalai Lama is one such person. He said, "I think this century will be a better century, a happier century."[1] While he acknowledges problems such as global warming and overpopulation, he remains hopeful, and recognizes that we are awakening at an amazingly accelerated rate.

Namaste. As we mentioned earlier, this is a Sanskrit word we say to each other at the end of every yoga class. One student recently told me, "To me, it's just a word, like peace." Yes, it is just a word, but a word that can change our world. *The Divine in me sees the Divine in you.* You are awake. I am awake.

The breezes at dawn have secrets to tell, don't go back to sleep!
You have to ask for what you really want, don't go back to sleep!
You know, there are those who go back and forth across the threshold, where
the two worlds meet, and the door, it's always open, and it's round, don't go
back to sleep.[2]
- Rumi

ᠭᠣ Practice Points

- Again, practice breathing consciously and deeply throughout the day to inspire presence and awareness. Move a bit more slowly and awaken to grace and life!

ᠭᠣ Contemplation: Intention to Awaken

- Connect with the breath, which invites presence.
- Make an intention--or prayer--for awakening. Express your willingness to be fully conscious.

GOD

There are hundreds of ways to kneel and kiss the ground.
- Rumi

Speaking of wakeup calls, here is a reminder for us all: You are God. I am God. Everyone and Everything is God.

Can it really be that simple, that reassuring? We *are* God? Perhaps, but at the same time God is the most unsettling, controversial, war-provoking topic on this planet. *My* God is better than *your* God. Or, there *is* no God. The word God is perhaps the most loaded word in our God-fearing world, so please feel free to replace it for the sake of this discussion. Alternatives include Source, Great Spirit, Allah, Universal Intelligence, or Divine Oneness--whatever works for you. Nonetheless, let's not avoid this tender topic.

Personally, I have had a strange love-hate relationship with my God. When I feel safe, and things are going my way, I may acknowledge God's presence, grace, and goodness. When I see a beautiful sunset I may say, "Oh my God." When I am raging, feeling alone, or stubbing my toe, my attitude changes to, "God darn it!"(or worse). How does God go from being my best friend to a royal jerk?

Perhaps you do not believe in God, or any god. Perfect. Yoga offers a respectful approach, which invites us to find our own clarity, although perhaps the yogis knew what we would find. I am told that many within the Hindu religion originally rejected the ideals of yoga because the early yogis refused to limit the yoga notion of *Ishvara*--the Divine, or Supreme--to the Hindi God or gods. Yoga does not deny these gods, nor does it endorse only certain gods or beliefs. Rather, yoga is about clearing the mind and finding your own truth, your own God, Goddess, or godlessness.

I have heard it said that we are either host to God, or hostage to ego. Dharma Mittra, a yoga teacher famous for his ability to stand on his head without the use of hands, along with hundreds of other incredible poses, says, "I don't encourage people to do fancy poses. They are not that important. The goal of yoga is Self-realization: to find out who you are, why you're here, who God is. God and the Self are the same--exactly the same."[1]

Let's have a little God-to-God talk. When you hear the word God, what do you think, or feel? What images arise? A personal, specific God or no god? Form, or formless? In man's image, or other? Perhaps you *feel* God when you gaze into a cloudless and silent starry night? Or when you walk barefoot on the Earth itself, or make love?

In some circles, it has become common to judge spirituality as better than religion, but religions are doing their best, and are imperfect like everything else in this world. Religions try to connect the populace, build community, study, and teach. Each of the religions is like a root of the same tree, seeking to tap into the Source and nourish the soul-branches. When fear and misunderstanding get in the way, however, separation, superiority, and control result. Organized religions, whether we are talking Christianity, Judaism, Islam, Mormonism, or Whateverism, sometimes misrepresent the supposed demands of God. Christianity is not alone in this, but its contradictions and strict moral requirements have resulted in control, denial, and domination of the body, emotions, and passions, resulting in the sexual crisis we see in many churches today.

Organized religions may have all started out with goodly- -or Godly--intentions, but have sometimes gotten lost in our human foibles, and have scared many of us away from the true nature of God. This is why many are leaving certain churches and organized religions and seeking their God on more personal or spiritual paths. Perhaps this is a healthy sign of an emerging new consciousness, where, rather than mold ourselves to a dogma, we trust ourselves and what makes sense to us.

We can release the *beliefs* and honor our heart's *knowing*. God is accessible right now, here, in the body. God is in the church and in the forest, in the East and of the West. While God is everywhere, we find God in our heart more easily than our head. In *Conversations with God*, Neale Donald Walsch says, "In order to truly know God, you have to be out of your mind."[2]

You and I and even the neighbors we don't like, are made up of the same stuff. We are like bits of the big package of God or Life Force, spread out as traces of universal intelligence, sometimes called souls. My God is the only God, and so is yours, for your God and my God are One.

This is good news. Since you, me, and everything else on the planet, in the universe, and beyond make up the countless aspects of God, then we Gods are creating our world. There is nothing or no one outside of ourselves to make rules, guide, control, or punish us and send us to hell. Again, there are consequences for our actions, but this is different from an external punishment. You might say that we punish or reward ourselves. If it's all God, then even that which we judge as bad or awful is actually *full of awe*. Thus, we constantly have the opportunity to see the Divine in our biggest challenges, whether they be enemies or tax collectors, hangovers or hemorrhoids.

If you and I are God, and we co-created this world, then we can recreate it. When we remember and reconnect with our inner God, and the Spirit within each and every person and animal and branch and stone, when we realize our essence, and have a change of heart, we will do godly things, and behave in saintly ways. This is what is referred to as Self-realization.

Let's not get lost in semantics. We can practice paying attention to that loving and always present inner voice. It is the God within, always patient, inviting, merciful. When we learn to distinguish and heed it above the chidings of fright, rivalry, and war, we have begun the wonderful process of healing our world. Let's not be afraid of any god, for there is nothing to fear. May you move forward, in the glory and power of the God-Goddess you truly are. As the Na'vi say in the Avatar movie: "I see you."

Only Breath

Not Christian or Jew or Muslim, not Hindu, Buddhist, Sufi, or Zen. Not any religion or cultural system. I am not from the East or the West, not out of the ocean or up from the ground . . . only that breath breathing human being.[3]
- Rumi

∞ Practice Points

- Are you ready for the ultimate practice? Can you practice seeing God in everyone and everything?
- Start where you can, perhaps with people, pets, or trees with which you already have an affinity. Then expand your practice…

⊛ **Contemplation: Connecting with God**

- Let the river of breath take you to the Source.
- Reflect on God (or your choice of word.) What feelings arise? Where did you first hear the word? Who taught you your idea of God? Move attention from the head to the heart and ask, what makes sense now? Ask God Himself--Herself. Ask your Self.

SACRED SERVICE

While there is a lower class, I am in it; while there is a criminal element, I am of it; while there is a soul in prison, I am not free.
- Eugene Victor Debbs

We are all in this together. We may fool ourselves with borders, gated communities, polarized political parties, and assorted languages and skin colors but we are truly beginning to grasp an understanding of our interconnectedness. While it is true that we must take care of ourselves, we must also take the same responsibility for each *other*. We find ourselves and expand ourselves when we give *of* ourselves.

I have known individuals and groups that are quite focused on the inner healing or spiritual journey, but unconcerned with the environmental or social justice issues in our "outer" world. And I have seen environmental or political activists who do not know themselves, and completely sidestep any spiritual questioning. And then there are those of us; myself included for many years--who avoid exploring the inner or outer landscapes, living narrow and mundane existences.

It's all okay, as we are all learning. The ideal, though, is a balance of inner-outer work, where we heal the world from the inside-out. We meditate, pray, or go to therapy, *and* we recycle, serve, or speak out. We take our expanded self into the world as a being of service. We can learn, as Andrew Harvey says, to "combine the wisdom of spiritual teachings with the passion of an activist."[1]

As we remember our relationship with everything and everyone, we no longer live with our small self in mind, but with our expanded Self in Mind. We use the gifts that we have, which were given to us not to personally enrich us, but to serve the greater good. Whether paid or unpaid, this is a sacred activism, the source of the joy and satisfaction we truly seek, being a part of, and doing our part in a thriving and connected community. As Krishna tells Arjuna in the *Bhagavad Gita*, "Strive constantly to serve the welfare of the world; by devotion to selfless work one attains the supreme goal of life."[2]

Intuitively, we all feel a longing to connect and serve, and on some level we all love to help. This instinct is alive and experienced the instant we hear about someone in need, or someone who is suffering. We get the gut level response--*how can I help*? When we disconnect from that feeling, we suffer. This genuine urge is what we feel when we come across a homeless person asking for a coin, although this empathy can be quickly squelched if we let the mind and ego jump in with their fearful chimes of separation: "I can't afford it," or "they don't deserve it."

With public service, we are saying, "You are as important as I am. You are worthy of respect. In fact, you *are* me." We step out of our little worlds. A healthy balance is what we seek, providing enough for ourselves without slipping into self-indulgence, and serving others without martyring ourselves and becoming bitter or depleted. What we give we get, and it is said that, "the fragrance stays in the hand that gives the flower."

We are all truly "socialists" in our heart of hearts. Part of us suffers knowing that as we eat our food, there are brothers and sisters who have to search for scraps. While some of us find it natural to buy new clothes or to live in a heated house, others are cold and homeless and cannot get their hands on basic necessities. At some point (or in some lifetime), we all find ourselves in need of a helping hand.

Many of us have a misguided belief that volunteer work has to be something painfully difficult. When we do what we love, it does not feel like work. Ideally, our best service, paid or not, is doing what gives us joy, sharing our gifts, so we feed the community and ourselves. Rather than heavy and draining, activism and service can be fulfilling. Just be you.

I have heard that the difference between a healthy empathy and an unhealthy empathy is like this: Say we are walking through the jungle and hear shouts for help, and see that someone is stuck in quicksand. The unhealthy reaction is to jump in to "save" the person, in which case both get sucked under. With compassion, we take a deep breath, keep our center, then respond by throwing a vine with which the person can pull *herself* free.

In the United States, we lack ritual. Perhaps we could implement some form of national community service as a rite of passage for our youth as they complete high school, or reach a certain age. Rather than urge them too quickly into an often self-serving career route before they really have a chance to know themselves, why not one year of public service? We could open up other options beyond the military to include environmental, peace, and various other social services. What a great transition this would be into adulthood and our community. Young people might become engaged, informed, and active world citizens, patriotic in a truly global or universal sense.

As we see in times of crisis, humans are givers and healers; the response is open-hearted compassion. We care about one another and we want to help. Aside from the rhetoric to consume and compete, deep down we know this is not who we are. While we are taught that the more money we make and stuff we acquire the happier we will be, some studies suggest that the more we *give away* or spend on *others*, the happier we feel.[3]

Learning to give is hard when we are struggling or suffering, but this is one way to both feel good and change our poverty mindset. Can we give back what we feel we lack? When we give, we are saying, "I have enough to share." If we presently cannot afford--or do not feel comfortable--giving materially or financially, we can practice giving compliments or smiles, as the energy is most important. This is an expression of the abundance of who we truly are: spiritual, limitless beings.

There is really only one way to become fulfilled and achieve joy and contentment: by giving those very things away, becoming a being of service. In the simplest of terms: *me* hurts and shrinks us. *We* heals and expands us.

Each time a person stands up for an ideal, or acts to improve the lot of others, or strikes out against injustice, he or she sends forth a tiny ripple of hope.[4]
 - Robert Kennedy

ᎶᎥ Practice Points

* Practice giving of yourself. Choose something that is doable (it can be time, compliments, money, etc.) Do you notice that when you give of yourself, you actually expand?

ᎶᎥ Contemplation: Sacred Service

* Reflect on times when you gave in service. How did this feel? How would you enjoy being of service?

LOVE AND COMPASSION

Know your Self and practice love and compassion.
 - Amma

When I think of love, I think of Amma. One spring day in 2005, I was having lunch with my friend Chris, who had recently been to a retreat with Amma, the Indian guru known as the "Hugging Saint." Chris was still absolutely glowing from the love she had experienced at that event. I then noticed that the rest of the day, I too felt vibrantly alive, just from being around Chris, who had been around Amma two days earlier! I knew I had to visit this Amma woman.

Two years later, I attended the annual Amma retreat weekend near Seattle, and I was not disappointed. This woman is pure love and compassion, and has hugged approximately 26 million people around the world. Her hug--called darshan--is a profoundly compassionate, motherly embrace. After each of her hugs, I felt blessed, blissed, and completely at ease. I found myself naturally drawn as close as possible to the *darshan* line, sitting and smiling for hours, bathing in the aura of love. Being a normally tense person, I was amazed at how little angst was left in my body--as if the pain plug had been pulled. Such is the power of love.

All of us have experienced love, in one of its many forms--romantic love, compassion, empathy, kindness--if only for precious fleeting moments. True love, ultimately, is the only energy that is deeply real, for love is the essence of who we are. Divine love is nothing like the superficial, transient human version, which can be selfish and rooted in personal needs and desires. Spiritual love is pure and unconditional. While the intellect and ego are sometimes limited in vision, our essential love is not blind, but sees beauty in everything.

Real love has no limits, although we often try to minimize it. One time, I was taking a woods walk with my friend Brian, who lives much of the year in Guatemala working with the highland Indians, running a wonderful project called Embrace Guatemala. At one point I casually asked, "So, with all this traveling, how is your love life?" He looked stunned, and then explained to me, "My *life* is love. The children I work with in Guatemala are full of love. I love the people in the villages, and I love my work." I had tried to compartmentalize love, or reduce it to the romantic realm, and Brian woke me up.

Another openhearted friend, Nancy, was in business school many years ago when she became frustrated and asked why ethics is not a mandatory college course for business majors. The answer she got was, "Ethics are already integrated into the business curriculum. You need to incorporate more head and less heart." In truth, we are wise to connect the head to the heart.

Love may be the greatest and perhaps only healer, the thread that underlies all true healing. No thing, nothing of this world, not fear or pain or anger or ignorance, can endure in its presence. When we let love in, everything else dissipates back into that which it came from--love. Jesus said, "There is no fear where love exists."[1]

Now, all this may sound like rubbish if we are currently experiencing hate or fear. Self-hate and other powerful emotions have a way of taking over and convincing us that they are more real and permanent than the supposedly lofty, dreamy, and distant realms of love and bliss. Love is often overshadowed by our internal turbulence, so our hearts close and we wall ourselves off. When we withhold love, we withhold our very selves, and we suffer.

Love cannot be explained, defined, or even understood on an intellectual level; it must be experienced. Fortunately, since it is our essential nature, we will. Love is always present; it just gets covered up, and the blankets of fear feel so real. Fortunately, at times grace may lift the fog and help us feel the aliveness: when holding a baby, petting a dog, or helping a friend in need.

The Dalai Lama tells us that we are biologically wired to compassionate care for one another; it is our nature. He also believes that women may have a greater gift of promoting compassion through their experience of mothering: "I think women should take a more important role in this age."[2]

Is there any word more healing than "love"? Is there anything we enjoy hearing more than "I love you"? Notice how you feel when you hear these words: *I love you.* In case you could not hear it or feel it, please take a deep breath, and allow me to repeat myself: *I love you.*

Consider that love is not something we have to seek, for it is here, now. As Amma says, "Love is our essential nature."[3] Be love, and be loved, for you are the beloved.

We have to remember that Mother Earth has a heart, that we should feel her energy, and send our thoughts of love.[4]
- Carlos Barrios

ൟ Practice Points

- Even when you do not feel it, see if you can practice loving kindness and compassion towards others, but especially towards yourself.

ൟ Contemplation: Om Mani Padme Hum (Behold the Jewel in the Lotus.)

This is a wonderful, powerful Sanskrit mantra in the Tibetan Buddhist tradition, used for expanding the Heart.

- Bring your attention to the heart chakra, in the middle of the chest.

- Imagine your favorite flower in the middle of your heart, with your favorite jewel within it.

- Silently--or out loud--begin to recite the mantra: *Om Mani Padme Hum* (sounds like om manee pod may hoom).

- Let the vibration of light and love blossom and reverberate through your entire body, into every cell, transforming the denser energies, leaving nothing but love.

- Beam this love out in every direction, filling every corner of the community, the nation, the planet. No effort, just allow the natural expression of who you are.

NATIVE WISDOM

Without love for the Earth there is no place for us in heaven.
- Aymara Oral Teachings

For much of modern history, Native peoples have been misunderstood and marginalized, and Native and ancient wisdom has been ignored or feared. This is changing, and now is the time to heal any rifts between Native peoples and those of us who have wandered from the way of the Earth. Chief Fools Crow (1890-1989) said, "Survival of the world depends on our sharing what we have, and working together."[1]

Phil Lane, Jr., head of the United Indians of all Tribes Foundation, says, "Indigenous people still have their hearts open to co-creating a sustainable, peaceful, harmonious future together."[2] Lane has spent his life helping others understand old prophecies that foretell a winter of suffering followed by a springtime of rebirth for Indigenous peoples. He mentions the many prophesies which talk of the northern Eagle and southern Condor tribes joining forces to take leadership roles in establishing world peace, social justice, and economic prosperity.

The Mayans, Aztecs, Hopis, and individual Native voices such as Black Elk went to great lengths to warn us about this period of tremendous transformation. Chief Seattle--once a leader of the Suquamish and Duwamish Native American tribes--ominously warned us back in the 1850s, "Contaminate your bed and you will one night suffocate in your own waste."[3] The Hopi prophecy warns of a time when earthquakes, storms, floods, drought, and famine become common, and signal the need to a return to the true path. The most common time mentioned is the around the end of the 5,125-year Mayan calendar on December 21, 2012.

It is important to know that this is not a one-day shift on December 21, 2012, although there is a specific alignment at that exact time. We are now in the midst of the change that is apparently lasting for several years before and after that date. Of course, this change is not only affecting what Native peoples call Turtle Island--North America--but the entire planet. Native Americans were not the only people to warn of the changes we are now experiencing. The biblical story of Revelation, the Hebrew Torah and its warning codes, the Vedas and other Hindu teachings all targeted this time as one of great change. The 8,000-year-old Hindu Vedic scriptures wrote of countless periods of birth and rebirth of the world. There is a consensus among many indigenous groups across the planet, from various places and time periods, that we are presently experiencing a time unlike any in recorded history.

Our modern scientists agree that our planets are moving into an extremely rare alignment. We are literally moving from an extended period of darkness, to a point where our solar system moves closer into alignment with the core of the Milky Way galaxy than it has been in about 26,000 years. While there are starry-eyed folks who say that there is nothing to worry about, others are declaring doomsday. Most of these ancient prophesies do not claim the end of the planet or humanity, although it appears likely that we will all be greatly affected by the upheaval.

I spoke to one Native elder named White Bear, from what we call the Apache tribe, who told me that this does not signify Armageddon or an end times event, not something to fear, but certainly something to take heed of and prepare for. He sees this as more of a spiritual shift. Of course, we all have some say in what kind of change occurs through our words, thoughts, feelings, and actions.

Do we continue the unsustainable way of war--on the Earth and on each other--or learn to work together?

Some Native people say this is the age of the White Buffalo, which also represents an era of transition and tremendous change. The birth of a white buffalo calf is seen by Native Americans as a prophetic symbol, a sign of mending of the sacred hoop, rebirth of Native wisdom, and world harmony. White Bear says that there are currently several white buffalo alive in North America.

Agnes Baker Pilgrim, a member of the very active International Council of Thirteen Indigenous Grandmothers, says, "The greatest distance in the world is the fourteen inches from our minds to our hearts."[4] This be a time of balancing the masculine right and feminine left wings. The Mayan elders of the Eagle Clan in Guatemala say this will be a fusion of both feminine and masculine energies, adding: "This is a cycle of wisdom, harmony, peace, love, of consciousness, and the return of the natural order. It is not the end of the world as many from outside of the Mayan tradition have misinterpreted it."[5]

Mayan Priest Carlos Barrios says, "We are coming closer to the end of the Four Ajaw, which is a cycle of 5,200 years that will end on December 20, 2012, and to the beginning of the Five Ajaw that will start on December 21, 2012. This date has been erroneously labeled as the "end of the world," which is a bad interpretation; it is the end of a cycle and the beginning of a new one that will bring the *Return to Awareness*, meaning it will be a cycle of spiritual development, of having the space to return to the natural order. This cycle brings us the opportunity to find a balance with Mother Earth and a harmonious relationship between the Feminine and the Masculine. It will be a period of light and wisdom that will bring a new economic and social order."[6]

While we humans are all indigenous inhabitants of this planet, and spiritual residents of our universe, there are those of us who have not lost their sacred Earth-Spirit roots. I pray that we recognize and honor these peoples and tribes who are helping us remember our sacred connections. With humility and openness, we can incorporate ancient wisdom, tradition, and sustainability, while infusing it with a new and vital vision and aliveness. May North and

South, East and West join together to create the best of all worlds, for we are the ones we have been waiting for.

ᏬᎥ Practice Points

* How can you apply Native wisdom to living in balance with the Earth, with concern for all our relations?

ᏬᎥ Contemplation: Earth Heartbeat

* Breathe deeply, open the heart, and connect with the Earth. Humbly ask for guidance, that you remember the way.
* Allow your heartbeat to match the pulse of the Earth.

HEALING

The message that underlies healing is simple yet radical: We are already whole.
- Joan Borysenko

Healing is awakening. Healing is simply remembering who we really are, resting in the assurance that we are already whole, always have been, and always will be.

Yet healing is accepting our humanity with humor and humility, along with all the inevitable imperfections and glitches that our living encompasses. The deepest healing is always accompanied by courage, for to step outside our story and let go of the familiar is neither easy nor comfortable. It is said that when we ask for polishing, we will be tumbled.

We are currently in the midst of one of our world's greatest "tumblings" of global consciousness, healing, and awakening, and so there is good news and bad news. With the quickening energy vibration and growing light, those who continue to close off their feelings will inevitably and increasingly suffer. Those who choose to take responsibility, face their darkness and denial, and declare their right to awaken will have ever more support and illumination to work with. Those who hold on will hurt, and those who let go will heal.

The Earth, which has been tremendously patient and accepting of our human presence, has reached a point where it must heal itself and balance out. It is doing this through the manifestation of disease, calamity, and other challenges of our day. As painful as this may be over the coming years, if we can keep breathing, stay grounded, and keep the long-range picture in mind, we can trust in the perfection of it all.

There are countless ideas on healing, many of which we have explored in this book. Some would say that healing is surrendering to universal principles or Spirit. Acceptance rather than judgment heals. Some say that healing is following our passion and power, doing what we are here to do. Perhaps healing is simply receiving a tender, well-timed embrace. Some might say that healing is finding a good therapist or listener who truly cares, who holds a space of compassion.

A good friend of mine, Laura, is a therapist and healer. She is present, kind, and a great listener. She sometimes feels like she does not do enough, but it is less *what we do* than *who we are.* After a recent session, a client paused, struggled for words, then looked directly at her, "I'm not sure what happens here, but something changes." That something is the Divine presence she invokes as the anchor for every session. She listens with love, and mirrors the person's own love and beauty back to them.

Some would say that the best thing a healer or therapist can do is simply love and be themselves, allow their own light and joy. The healer knows she is not responsible for healing. She gets ego out of the way and allows space for grace, knowing that compassionate, unattached presence is key.

We are learning how to heal. We are moving away from a curative, downstream, disease-oriented approach to a preventative, upstream, holistic model. By 2009, Americans were spending about $35 billion a year on various alternative therapies which were not covered by insurance plans. We are returning to and re-learning ancient secrets and wisdom. Western medicine is still valuable; when we break a leg, we may not first choose someone to administer tea tree oil--we go to a hospital. We are integrating all we know.

At times healing is a mystery, but not magical. It is simply acknowledging the wounds, while reminding ourselves of who we are, recognizing that we are so much bigger than our emotions and pains. Sometimes when I mention healing, people look confused, as if to say, "I'm fine, there's nothing wrong with me that needs healing." Of course, they are right. Yet while we are holy and whole, our humanity suffers, poverty is widespread, wars continue, and the Earth is on fire. On a very human level, we are half-alive, we all have healing to do, and denial is the antithesis of healing.

As we move out of denial, when we bravely or even desperately decide to enter into our wounds, we need not live there, over-evaluating, dredging up every hint of evidence about our mistreatment, sticking to the story. We visit it to heal it. The Buddha reportedly said, "When felled by an arrow, are you going to quarrel about its origins, or pull it out?"[1]

Healing is presence, coming fully home to your personal body and anchoring into the Earth, paying attention to yourself, each other, and your God. Healing is dancing to the natural rhythms of the planet, making love, petting the cat, or walking the dog. Healing is laughing when there is nothing left to do.

Healing is yin and yang, surrendering and asserting. Healing is building community even when we feel like running and hiding in some cave and never coming out. And healing is taking some time in the cave to renew and find ourselves. Healing is emptying and therefore filling. Healing is voice and expression, stillness and silence. For one, healing is praying with the rosary, while another chanting a Vedic verse with incense or candles gracing a sacred space. For another, healing is letting another cut in line at the grocery store, or paying their bill. Healing is giving and serving, and receiving and asking for help.

Healing may be simply stopping doing what is harmful, or doing whatever breaks the cycle and attachment to pain and disease. I hear that our bodies create 300 million new cells every minute-- of course, we can change and are changing! We heal when we envision or can allow something new. Brooke Medicine Eagle said, "Anything can be used that, without causing damage or unnecessary distress, creates a radical discontinuity in the way the dis-eased person's reality is assembled. Then the dance toward wholeness can begin."[2]

Above all, this book is an invitation and encouragement to practice the art of healing through compassionate presence and self-love. Religious scholar Karen Armstrong, in all her extensive studies of world religions, says that one thing came up repeatedly, "Compassion was the major test of any true spirituality . . ."[3] The holy book of the Muslim faith, the Qu'ran (also translated as Koran) cites the following words one hundred and ninety-two times, starting nearly every chapter: "In the name of Allah, infinitely compassionate, infinitely merciful."

If you can take one thing from this book, a good choice would be this: have merciful compassion for yourself. For being human is difficult, and compassion is the balm that soothes our aches and eases the struggle. Self-love is our ultimate practice. The 17th Karmapa from Tibet says, "Kindness is the most important thing."[4]

The words and many sections and suggestions in this book--grounding, feeling, creating community, never giving up-- are all simply reminders and stepping stones. But remember that in a moment we can leap over them and know the truth and depth of our love, here, now. Healing is remembering: we are that which we seek.

೫ Practice Points

- Practice allowing each of your daily 15,000 breaths to be full, easy, and natural.

೫ Contemplation: Receiving Merciful Compassion

- Ask the universe or Spirit for gracious, compassionate healing, and allow your body to receive and fill with light. Feel merciful self-compassion.

LIGHTEN UP

I arise in the morning torn between a desire to improve the world and a desire to enjoy the world.
- E.B. White

All this personal and global healing work can be exhausting! If you are anything like me, you've gotten so tired of pain and so desperate to relieve--rather than re-live--the despair and depression, that you are doing anything and everything to rid yourself of it.

I went on a comprehensive personal healing spree that lasted many years, from tai chi and hypnotherapy to raw foods and fasting to psychotherapy and Rolfing. While I have no regrets, some of this work was expensive and unnecessary. Furthermore, my compulsive healing sometimes furthered my confusion, deepened my depression, and distracted me from simply being fully present for much of this rich and valuable experience. I was often trying so hard to be anywhere but present, that I could not grasp the beauty of the moment. And all of the journey--the pain, the fear, the depression--*is* beautiful.

In the earlier chapter "Come Home," we looked at the need to come back to the body. Well, we do not have to inhabit every room and clean the whole house in one swoop. In fact, when we start the healing path and face the daunting goal of awakening from our sleep, we don't know where to start. Like spring-cleaning, we can start with one closet, or one deep breath.

We are already whole! We can stop trying so hard to heal, and just lighten up. We adults are forgetting how to laugh, be silly, and have fun. Studies show that children can laugh 300-400 times a day, but by adulthood, it is down to 15--on a good day![1] There is an Oriental proverb: "Time spent laughing is time spent with the gods."

It is said that we all laugh and cry in the same language. One day, I was sitting on a beach in Australia with two friends, an American named Chris Brady, and a British guy named Mike Clark, who had that wonderful British wit. Chris and I had this habit of using this word *schmutz*, which we loosely translated as anything from getting tipsy on Australian beers (schmutzed--which we did lots of at that time) or stepping in some dog poop--schmutz! One moment, Mike interrupted me, asking, "Schmutz, schmutz--you guys always use this word--what does "schmutz" mean anyway?" At that very moment, a seagull passed over, dropping a gooey glob right on top of Mike's head. Without expression or hesitation, he calmly reached up, touched the top of his head, and said, "Oh, schmutz."

I have heard that God is a standup comic, but his audience is too afraid to laugh. Healing work can be schmutzy, bewildering, and amusing. But our *crap* is our manure for growth. Only pride keeps us from just letting go and admitting that we do not have it all together. Does anyone?

Humor is also very attractive. Studies show that a sense of humor is one of the best traits for attracting a mate. So at the least, humor may attract some friends for the journey. And laughter itself may pull us out of depression or pain--at least for a moment. I have an easy way to tell when I am out of whack--I lose my sense of humor (although I'm often too serious to recognize it). If we keep our wit, we have our sanity and spirit.

Anyone who takes themselves too seriously is probably further from truth than they realize. One of the first things I look for in a healer or teacher or spiritual group is humor. If they are too serious, they are generally not for me. This is not to say that all teachers and healers have to be funny--we all have different gifts. But if they have a hint of humor, it helps me take them, well, seriously.

Please use anything from this book that feels helpful, and release the rest. Feel the sense of urgency on Earth at this time, yes, but do so with a spiritual softness, an easy breath, and a light and open heart.

"When you realize how perfect everything is you will tilt your head back and laugh at the sky."[2]
- The Buddha

⊙ Practice Points

* Can you lighten up today? Can you do something fun or silly?

⊙ Contemplation: None

* No meditation homework today--goof off!

CONCLUSION

There is no conclusion, only the ever-continuing dance of life itself, of cycles and spirals, of birth and death. Be, breathe, play, laugh, see, feel, and heal. Be human, yet do so divinely. Be your Self, for you are great and beautiful, and your presence, power, and passion are so needed at this tremendous time of transition on planet Earth.

My current feeling regarding the Earth changes is this. Physically, the challenges will almost certainly intensify for awhile, and many of us may not make it much further--at least in these bodies. We can never be attached to anything, especially at this time: our relationships, our careers-even our bodies and lives themselves.

Spiritually, all is perfect, for we are everlasting beings. Life moves in cycles, and the good news right now is that we appear to be leaving the darkest days and heading into a world age, or yuga, of increasing consciousness and expanding light. I hope and sense this to be true, and I am honored to be with you at this amazing time on Earth.

May you be present and open to each and every magnificent mystery, and even the momentary misery! I bless you and your journey. I honor you. I bow to you.

Inlakesh! Mayan greeting which means "We are different faces of each other."

Notes

The bibliography is arranged by parts and chapters, in the exact order in which they appear in the book.

Part One: Presence

Breath by Breath
1. Iyengar, B.K.S., *Light on Life*, with John J. Evans and Douglas Abrams, Rodale, 2005, p. 66.
2. Kraftsow, Gary, *Yoga for Wellness*, Penguin Compass, 1999, p. 306.
3. Rumi, Jelaluddin, *The Essential Rumi*, Translated by Coleman Barks, HarperSanFrancisco, 1995, p. 52. Translation of Jelaluddin Rumi by Neil Douglas-Klotz from The Sufi Book of Life: Ninety-nine Pathways of the Heart for the Modern Dervish, (Penguin Putnam, 2005). Copyright Neil Douglas-Klotz 2005. Reprinted with permission. Abwoon Resource Center www.abwoon.com

Pay Attention
Epigraph: Shabkar, *Offerings, Buddhist Wisdom for Every Day,* Oliver & Danielle Föllmi, Stewart, Tabori & Chang, New York, 2003, back page.

Come Home
Epigraph: Kabir, in *Wherever You Go There You Are,* Jon Kabat-Zinn, Hyperion, 1994, p. 60.
1. Kabir, *in Wherever You Go There You Are,* Jon Kabat-Zinn, Hyperion, 1994, p. 97.

Are You Out of Your Mind?
Epigraph: Berra, Yogi, *Meditation For Dummies,* Stephan Bodian, IDG Books Worldwide, 1999, p. 288.

Silence, Slowness, and Space
Epigraph: Hafiz, Persian Poet and Sufi master, *The Gift,* translation by Daniel Ladinsky, Penguin Compass, 1999, Preface.
1. Author Lin Yutang, *The Week,* August 19, 2005, p. 19.
2. Chief Seattle, *Critical Path,* R. Buckminster Fuller, St. Martin's Press, 1981, p. 65.
3. Rumi, Jelaluddin, *The Essential Rumi,* Translated by Coleman Barks, HarperSanFrancisco, 1995, p. 69.

Know Yourself
Epigraph: Muhammad, *Hadith,* in *The Fragrance of Faith,* by Jamal Rahman, The Book Foundation, 2004, p. 31.
1. _____. *AARP Bulletin,* June 2007, p.3.
2. _____. *AARP Bulletin,* June 2007, p.3.
3. *The Bhagavad Gita* 5:16, Translated by Eknath Easwaran, with chapter introductions by Diana Morrison, Shambhala, Boston & London, 2004, p. 121.

4. *A Course in Miracles*, Foundation for Inner Peace, 1992, p. 14.

Look Within
Epigraph: Voice of God heard by Neale Donald Walsch, *Conversations with God, Book 1*, G.P. Putnam's Sons, 1995, p. 44.
1. The Yoga Sutra 1.21, Chip Hartranft, The *Yoga Sutras of Patanjali*, Shambhala, Boston & London, 2003, p.98.
2. *A Course in Miracles*, Foundation for Inner Peace, 1992, p. 18.

Being You: Truth and Authenticity
Epigraph: Shakespeare, William, *Hamlet*, act I, scene iii, lines 78–80. Polonius is speaking to Laertes, Columbia Encyclopedia.
1. Paramhansa Yogananda, *The Autobiography of a Yogi*, Paramhansa Yogananda, Crystal Clarity Publishers, 1946, p. 228.
2. Jesus, *New American Standard Bible*, John 8:32, 1995.

Meditation and Prayer
Epigraph: Jesus, *King James Bible*, Psalm 46:10.
1. _____. Weiner, Eric, *The Week*, September 28, 2007, p.14.
2. Rumi, Jelaluddin, *The Essential Rumi*, Translated by Coleman Barks, HarperSanFrancisco, 1995, p. 35.

Part Two: Body and Emotions

Love and Move your Body
Epigraph: _____. Adams, Joey, *The Week*, June 29, 2007, p. 17.
1. Paramhansa Yogananda, *The Autobiography of a Yogi*, Paramhansa Yogananda, Crystal Clarity Publishers, 1946, p. 266.

Yogaaahhhhhhhhh . . .
Epigraph: *The Bhagavad Gita*, Translated by Eknath Easwaran, Shambhala Press, 1985, p. 114.
1. Ram Gopal, in *The Autobiography of a Yogi*, Paramhansa Yogananda, Crystal Clarity Publishers, 1946, p. 138.

Food and Nutrition
Epigraph: LaLane, Jack, *Natural Cures They Don't Want You to Know About*. By Kevin Trudeau, Published by Westview Press, 2007, p. 77.
1. _____. *Alternative Therapies in Health and Medicine*, July/August 2005.
2. _____. *Time Magazine*, June 4, 2007, p. 14.

Be an Animal
Epigraph. _____. *The Week*, January 11, 2008, p. 35.
1. Butler, Samuel, *The Way of All Flesh*, E.P. Dutton and Company, New York, 1916, p.92.

Be a Child
Epigraph: Jesus, *International Standard Version Bible*, Matthew 18:3.
1. _____. *The Herald, Little Miss Make-a-Difference*, Amy Daybert, October 23, 2009 p. B1-2.

2. Amma, *Embracing the World: Images and Sayings of Sri Mata Amritanandamayi Devi*, Mata Amritanandamayi Mission Trust, September 2003, p. 36.

3. Kataria, Dr. Madan, *Laugh for No Reason*, Madhuri International, 1999, p. 12.

4. Kornfield, Jack, *The Wise Heart,* A Bantam Book, 2008, p. 395.

Create Community

Epigraph: Jesus, *New Revised Standard Edition Bible*, Matthew 18:20.

1. The 14th Dalai Lama, heard at public appearance at Qwest Stadium, Seattle, April 12, 2008.

2. Carnegie, Dale, in T.D. Jakes book, *He-Motions,* G.P. Putnam's Sons, member of Penguin Group (USA) Inc., Copyright T.D. Jakes, 2004, p. 146.

Feeling Feelings

Epigraph: Rumi, Jelaluddin, *The Guest House,* in *The Essential Rumi,* Translated by Coleman Barks, HarperSanFrancisco, 1995, p. 109.

1. Hartranft, Chip, *The Yoga Sutras of Patanjali,* Shambhala, Boston & London, 2003, p. 154.

2. Brennan, Barbara Ann, *Hands of Light, A Guide to Healing Through the Human Energy Field,* A Bantam Book, 1987, p. 99.

Allowing Anger

Epigraph: Blake, William, Online text © 2003, Ian Lancashire for the Department of English, University of Toronto. Published by the Web Development Group, Information Technology Services, University of Toronto Libraries.

Fear Not

Epigraph: Jesus, John 14:27, *Jesus and Buddha,* Marcus Borg, Ulysses Press, 1997, p. 82.

1. Keller, Helen, *Time for Joy: Daily Affirmations*. By Ruth Fishel, Bonny Van de Kamp. Illustrated by Bonny Van de Kamp. Published by HCI, 1998, p. 146.

2. O'Keeffe, Georgia, *ConZentrate: Get Focused and Pay Attention--When Life Is Filled with Pressures, Distractions, and Multiple Priorities*. By Sam Horn, Published by Macmillan, 2001, p. 296.

3. King, Jr., Rev. Martin Luther, on the eve of his assassination, Memphis Tennessee, April 3, 1968, in *The Martin Luther King, Jr. Companion,* Selected by Coretta Scott King, St. Martin's Press, N.Y., 1993, p. 99.

Part Three: Balance and Open Mindedness

Making Peace with Paradox

Epigraph: Kornfield, Jack, *A Path with Heart,* A Bantam Book, 1993, p. 27.

1. _____. Laptides, Beth, *LAYOGA*, November 2009, Volume 8, no. 9, p. 22.

Yin: Patience and Surrender

Epigraph: Amma, *Conscious Choice Seattle,* a Conscious Enlightenment Publication, June 2006, p. 35.

1. Lao-Tzu, in Jon Kabat Zinn, *Wherever You Go There You Are,* Hyperion. 1994, p. 51.

Yang: Action and Assertiveness

Epigraph: Jesus, in Matthew, 18:15, *The Method And Message of Jesus' Teachings,* by Robert H. Stein, Published by Westminster John Knox Press, 1994, p. 11.

Forgive and Let Go

1. Carter, Rubin, *Hurricane, The Miraculous Journey of Rubin Carter,* James S. Hirsch, Mariner Books / Houghton Mifflin Company, 2000 p. 310.
2. Jesus, *King James Version King James Bible,* Luke 23:34.
3. Wiener, Richard, Power of Forgiveness Workshop, 5/3/09, by permission of Richard Wiener.

Acceptance and Non-judgment

Epigraph: Epictetus, *Wisdom of the Ages,* by Dr. Wayne W. Dyer, Harper Collins, 1998, p. 31.

1. *A Course in Miracles,* Foundation for Inner Peace, 1992, p. 65.
2. Kornfield, Jack, *A Path with Heart,* A Bantam Book, 1993, p. 47.
3. Dalai Lama, *The Wise Heart: Guide to the Universal Teachings of Buddhist Psychology,* by Jack Kornfield, Random House, Inc., 2009, p. 391.

Nonattachment and Nonresistance

Epigraph: Maharishi, Ramana, in *Inspiration, Your Ultimate Calling,* by Dr. Wayne W. Dyer, Hay House, Inc., 2006, p. 71.

Faith and Trust

Epigraph: Cohen, Alan, (in email newsletter; received permission via internet communication).

1. Einstein, Albert, *Attitudes of Gratitude. How to Give and Receive Joy Every Day of Your Life, Mary Jane Ryan, Conari, 2009, p. 77.*
2. Mandela, Nelson, *Wisdom for the Soul of Black Folk*, Larry Chang, Roderick Terry, Gnosophia Publishers, 2007, p. 258.
3. Roy, Arundhati, Spoken at World Social Forum, in *Ecology, Economy, and God: Theology that Matters,* by Darby Kathleen Ray, Published by Fortress Press, 2006, p.188.

New Perspectives

Epigraph: O'Hara, J.T., *The Sun,* July 2003, Issue 331.

1. Thoreau, Henry David, *The Wildlife Companion,* by Malcolm Tait, Contributor Malcolm Tait, Published by Anova Books, 2004, p 107.
2. Kabat-Zinn, Jon, *Wherever You Go There You Are,* Hyperion, 1994.

Challenge Your Beliefs

Epigraph: *A Course in Miracles,* Foundation for Inner Peace, 1992, p.131.

1. Wordsworth, William, *Inspiration, Your Ultimate Calling*, by Dr. Wayne W. Dyer, Hay House, Inc., 2006, p. 157.
2. Gilbert, Geoffrey, *Rich and Poor in America:* A Reference Handbook, Published by ABC-CLIO, 2008, p. 8.
3. _____. Swift, Jonathan, *The Week*, September 23, 2005, p. 21.
4. _____. King, Larry, *Time Magazine*, June 1, 2009, p. 4.

Mystery and Humility

Epigraph: Rumi, Jelaluddin, *The Essential Rumi*, Translated by Coleman Barks, HarperSanFrancisco, 1995, p. 16.
1. Jesus, Luke 14:11, *New International Bible*, 1984.
2. Suzuki, Shunryu, *Zen Mind, Beginner's Mind*, Edited by Trudy Dixon, Shambhala Publications, 2006, p. 40.
3. Milarepa, *Offerings, Buddhist Wisdom for Every Day*, May 29, Oliver & Danielle Föllmi, Stewart, Tabori & Chang, New York, 2003.

Part Four: Energy

Grounding

Epigraph: Judith, Anodea, *Eastern Body Western Mind: Psychology and the Chakra System*, Celestial Arts Publishing 1996, p. 54.

Chakras

Epigraph: Judith, Anodea, *Eastern Body Western Mind: Psychology and the Chakra System*, Celestial Arts Publishing 1996, p. 6.

Life Force Energy

Epigraph: _____. Swami Veda Bharati, *LA Yoga–Ayurveda and Health Magazine*, June 2008, p. 40.

Imagine That

Epigraph: The Buddha, in *Awaken the Giant Within: How to Take Immediate Control of Your Mental, Emotional, Physical and Financial Destiny!* Anthony Robbins, Free Press, a Division of Simon and Schuster, 1991, p. 92.
1. Einstein, Albert, in *Awaken the Giant Within: How to Take Immediate Control of Your Mental, Emotional, Physical and Financial Destiny!* Anthony Robbins, Free Press, a Division of Simon and Schuster, 1991, p. 402.
2. Cohen, Alan, (email newsletter; received permission via internet communication).
3. _____. Yunus, Muhammad, *Time Magazine*, October 19, 2009, p.

Gratitude

Epigraph: Rumi, Jelaluddin, in Jack Kornfield, *A Path with Heart*, A Bantam Book, 1993, p. 335.
1. Jesus, *New American Standard Bible*, 1995.
2. _____. *ODE magazine*, email July, 24, 2007.

Boundaries

Epigraph: Brennan, Barbara Ann, *Light Emerging, The Journey of Personal Healing,* Bantam Books, 1993, p. 9.

1. _____. Amma, *Conscious Choice Seattle,* a Conscious Enlightenment Publication, Rod Sidon, June 2006.

Do Unto Others

Epigraph: The Beatles, *The End,* on *Abbey Road* album, credited to Lennon/McCartney. Produced by George Martin, 1969.

1. Jesus, *King JamesKing James Bible Bible,* Matthew 7:12.

2. Kabat-Zinn, Jon, *Wherever You Go There You Are,* Hyperion, 1994, p. 64.

3. Ihaleakala Hew Len, PhD., *Ho'oponopono prayer,* heard by Saul Maraney--permission granted on his website.

Simplicity

Epigraph: Wu-men, in Jon Kabat-Zinn, *Wherever You Go There You Are,* Hyperion, 1994, p. 16.

1. Sitting Bull, *The Cambridge History of American Literature,* Cambridge University Press, Edited by Sacvan Bercovitch, 1994, p.535.

2. Keller, Helen, *The Book of Uncommon Quips and Quotations.* By Venkata Ramana, Published by Pustak Mahal, 2004, p. 42.

Sacred Space

Epigraph: Bombeck, Erma, *The Subtlety of Emotions.* By Aharon Ben-Ze'ev, Published by MIT Press, 2000, p. 131.

1. _____. *ODE magazine,* Nov/Dec, 2009, Volume 7, Issue 8, p.36.

2. Gandhi, Mohandas K., *Peace and Conflict Studies,* 2nd Edition, David P. Barash and David P. Webel, Sage Publications, Inc, 2008, p. 459.

3. Frank, Anne, *The Book of Positive Quotes,* 2nd Edition, Compiled and arranged by John Cook, Fairview Press, 2007, p. 157.

4. Gandhi, Mohandas K., *Josephine, In Her Words: Our Mom.* By Tuchy Palmieri. Published by Carl (Tuchy) Palmieri, 2007, p. 110.

5. Einstein, Albert, *Nature, the End of Art: Environmental Landscape,* By Alan Sonfist, Wolfgang Becker, Robert Rosenblum, Published by D.A.P., 2004, p. 163.

Part Five: Peace with Pain

Earth Challenges

Epigraph: Hogan, Linda, *The Creation Spirit,* Andrea Skevington, Lion Pub UK, 2009, p. 9.

1. _____. Walsch, Neale Donald, *Everything is Changing—Are you Ready? Evolve,* Volume 8, Number 3, p. 14.

2. _____. *Time Magazine,* November 16, 2009, International Union for Conservation of Nature, 2009 Red List, p.14.

3. Chopra, Deepak, *Peace is the Way,* 2005, Three Rivers Press, p. 102

4. Perez, Don Alejandro Cirilo, Return of the Ancestors Gathering, YouTube, January 11, 2009.

Radical Responsibility

Epigraph: Tolle, Eckhart, *The Power of Now, A Guide to Spiritual Enlightenment*, New World Library, 1999, p. 65.
1. Gandhi, *Making of the Mahatma*, Raojobhai M. Patel, Published by Ravindra R. Patel, Copyright: Prashant R. Patel, 1990, p. 58.
2. _____. *The Week*, November 20, 2009, p. 20.
3. Perez, Don Alejandro Cirilo, Return of the Ancestors Gathering, YouTube, January 11, 2009.

Make Use of Suffering

Epigraph: Amiel, Henri-Frédéric, *Shoot the Damn Dog, A Memoir of Depression*, Sally Brampton, 2008, p. 1.
1. Krisnamacharya, *The Heart of Yoga*, T.K.V. Desikachar, Inner Traditions International, 1999, p. 146.
2. Thoreau, Henry David, *Walden: Or, Life in the Woods*, Francis Henry Allen. Published by Houghton Mifflin Co., 1910, p. 8.
3. Mirdad, Michael, *Evolve*, Volume 8, Number 3, P. 6.
4. Bodian, Stephan, *Meditation For Dummies*, IDG Books Worldwide, 1999, p. 83.

Learn from Failure and Challenge

Epigraph: Edison, Thomas, *Patent It Yourself*, 13th Edition, David Pressman, NOLO Publisher, 2008, p. 39.
1. _____. Obama, Barack, *Time Magazine, FDR's Lessons for Obama*, David M. Kennedy, July 6, 2009, p.29.
2. _____. Jordan, Michael, *Ode Magazine*, October 2008, p. 44.
3. Kornfield, Jack, *A Path with Heart*, A Bantam Book, 1993, p. 71.
4. Rumi, Jelaluddin, *The Essential Rumi*, Translated by Coleman Barks, HarperSanFrancisco, 1995, p. 3.

Relationships as Mirrors

Epigraph: Ford, Debbie, *The Dark Side of the Light Chasers*, Riverhead Books, 1998, p. 62.
1. Jesus, *The Method and Message of Jesus' Teachings*, By Robert H. Stein, Published by Westminster John Knox Press, 1994, p. 11.

Making Peace with Pain

Epigraph: Bradshaw, John, in *Eastern Body Western Mind*, Anodea Judith, Celestial Arts Publishing, 1996, p. 154.
1. Voice of God heard by Neale Donald Walsch, *Conversations with God, Book 1*, G.P. Putnam's Sons, 1995, p. 100.

Addictions

Epigraph: Emmons, Nathaniel, in *Awaken the Giant Within: How to Take Immediate Control of Your Mental, Emotional, Physical and Financial Destiny!* Anthony Robbins, Free Press, A Division of Simon and Schuster, 1991, p. 309.
1. _____. *AARP Bulletin, My English Teacher's Admonition*, Editor Jim Toedtman, January-February 2010, p. 3.
2. National Institute of Mental Health, *The Numbers Count: Mental*

Illness in America, Science on Our Minds Fact Sheet Series, January 15, 2005.

3. _____. *The Week,* AP investigation, Sept 7, 07, p. 23.

Depression and Grief

Epigraph: Bodian, Stephan, *Meditation For Dummies,* IDG Books Worldwide, 1999, p 277.

1. _____. *The Week,* AP investigation, September 7, 2007, p. 23.

2. _____. *The Week, Antidepressants: Costly Placebo?,* January 22, 2010, p. 19.

3. _____. *The Week, The world's most depressed nation,* Bret Stephens, March 23, 2007, p. 26.

4. _____. Harris Interactive and RightNow Technologies, *The Week,* November 2006, p. 48.

5. *A Course in Miracles,* Foundation for Inner Peace, 1992, p. 151.

6. Cowper, William, *The Poetical Works of William Cowper,* William Cowper, William Benham, MacMillan, 1908, p. 120.

Never Give up

Epigraph: Rumi, Jelaluddin, *The Essential Rumi,* Translated by Coleman Barks, HarperSanFrancisco, 1995, p. 64.

1. Churchill, Winston, *Stay Confident,* By John Caunt, Published by Kogan Page Publishers, 2001, p. 21.

2. University of British Columbia, *Human Security Report 2005: War and Peace in the 21ˢᵗ Century, 2005.*

3. The 14th Dalai Lama, *Wisdom for a High School Grad: Incredible Letters and Inspiring Advice for Getting the Most Out of College,* By Douglas Barry, Published by Running Press, 2005, p. 139.

Own Your Dark Side

Epigraph: Gandhi, Mohandas K., in *The Dark Side of the Light Chasers,* Debbie Ford, Riverhead Books, 1998, p. 176.

1. Solzhenitsyn, Aleksandr, in *The Wise Heart, A Guide to the Universal Teachings of Buddhist Psychology,* Kornfield, Jack, Bantam Books 2008, p. 155.

2. *A Course in Miracles,* Foundation for Inner Peace, 1992, p. 11.

3. Lao Tzu, *Tao te Ching, An Illustrated Journey,* translated by Stephen Mitchell, Frances Lincoln ltd, 1999, p. 1.

4. King, Jr., Rev. Martin Luther, in *The Martin Luther King, Jr. Companion,* Selected by Coretta Scott King, St. Martin's Press, N.Y., 1993, p. 56.

Part Six: Power, Purpose and Passion

Own Your Light Side

Epigraph: Rumi, Jelaluddin, *The Essential Rumi,* Translated by Coleman Barks, HarperSanFrancisco, 1995, p. 20.

Illuminating the Illusions

Epigraph: *A Course in Miracles*, Foundation for Inner Peace, 1992, p. 18.

1. *Webster's Dictionary and Thesaurus*, Geddes & Grosset, David Dale House, 2002, p. 186.
2. The 14th Dalai Lama, *Offerings, Buddhist Wisdom for Every Day*, May 8, Oliver & Danielle Föllmi, Stewart, Tabori & Chang, New York, 2003.
3. Rumi, Jelaluddin, *The Essential Rumi*, Translated by Coleman Barks, HarperSanFrancisco, 1995, p. 32.
4. Iyengar, B.K.S., Preface, *Light on Life,* with John J. Evans and Douglas Abrams, Rodale 2005, Preface.

Commitment to *Your* Path

Epigraph: Von Goethe, Johann Wolfgang, in *Awaken the Giant Within: How to Take Immediate Control of Your Mental, Emotional, Physical and Financial Destiny!* Anthony Robbins, Free Press, a Division of Simon and Schuster, 1991, p. 38.

1. Emerson, Ralph Waldo, *Worth Repeating*, Bob Kelly, Kregel Publications 2003, p. 108.
2. _____. Van Dyke, Henry, *The Week*, November 6, 2009, p. 21.

Power Up!

Epigraph: Chardin, Pierre Teilhard de, *Experiential Drawing,* by Robert Regis Dvorak, Published by Thomson Crisp Learning, 1991, p. 103.

1. _____. Lappé, Frances Moore, *Conscious Choice Seattle,* a Conscious Enlightenment Publication, August 2007, p. 36.
2. Jesus, *The Holy Bible, John, 12:14.*
3. Emerson, Ralph Waldo, in *Inspiration, Your Ultimate Calling,* by Dr. Wayne W. Dyer, Hay House, Inc., 2006, p. 64.
4. Clarke, Arthur C., in *Awaken the Giant Within: How to Take Immediate Control of Your Mental, Emotional, Physical and Financial Destiny!* Anthony Robbins, Free Press, a Division of Simon and Schuster, 1991, p. 409.

Wake Up!

Epigraph: Rinpoche, Chögyam Trungpa, *Places that Scare You: A Guide to Fearlessness in Difficult Times*, by Pema Chodron, Published by Shambhala, 2002, p. 89.

1. The 14th Dalai Lama, Heard at speech at Qwest Field, Seattle, April 12, 2008.
2. Rumi, Jelaluddin, *The Essential Rumi*, Translated by Coleman Barks, HarperSanFrancisco, 1995, p. 36.

God

Epigraph: Rumi, Jelaluddin, *The Essential Rumi*, Translated by Coleman Barks, HarperSanFrancisco, 1995, p. 36.

1. _____. Mittra, Dharma, *Yoga + Joyful Living*, March-April 2008, p. 55.
2. Voice of God heard by Neale Donald Walsch, *Conversations with*

God, Book 1, G.P. Putnam's Sons, 1995, p. 94.
3. Rumi, Jelaluddin, *The Essential Rumi,* Translated by Coleman Barks, HarperSanFrancisco, 1995, p. 32.

Sacred Service

Epigraph: Debbs, Eugene Victor, in *Awaken the Giant Within: How to Take Immediate Control of Your Mental, Emotional, Physical and Financial Destiny!* Anthony Robbins, Free Press, A Division of Simon and Schuster, 1991, p. 496.
1. _____. Harvey, Andrew, *Your Guide to Sacred Activism, Yoga+Joyful Living,* Winter 2009-10, p. 36.
2. Krishna, *Bhagavad Gita,* Translated by Eknath Easwaran, Shambhala Press 1985, p. 100.
3. _____. *How to Buy Happiness*, *The Week,* April 11, 2008, p. 22.
4. _____. Kennedy, Robert, *Your Guide to Sacred Activism, Yoga+Joyful Living,* Winter 2009-10, p. 40.

Love and Compassion

Epigraph: _____. Amma, *Conscious Choice Seattle,* a Conscious Enlightenment Publication, June 2006, p. 35.
1. Jesus, *International Standard Version Bible,* John 4:18.
2. The 14th Dalai Lama, heard in person, QWest Stadium, April 12, 2008.
3. Amma, *Embracing the World: Images and Sayings of Sri Mata Amritanandamayi Devi,* Mata Amritanandamayi Mission Trust, September 2003, p. 38.
4. Mayan Priest Carlos Barrios, *The New Humanity On The New Earth*, Hopi Newsletter Techqua Ikachi, August 30, 2008, with permission from Bill Tenuto.

Native Wisdom

Epigraph: Aymara oral teachings
1. Chief Fools Crow, Ceremonial Chief/Healer of the Teton Lakota band, *Fools Crow: Wisdom and Power,* Thomas E. Mails, Council Oak Books, 2001, p. 18.
2. Lane, Jr., Phil, CEO of the United Indians of all Tribes Foundation, *United Indians Website,* http://www.unitedindians.org/
3. Chief Seattle, Simulacrum America: *The USA and the Popular Media,* Edited by Elisabeth Kraus, Carolin Auer, Camden House, 2000, p. 162
4. _____. Pilgrim, Agnes Baker, *Grannies with a Mission, ODE Magazine,* Jan/Feb 2010, Volume 8, Issue 1, p. 63.
5. The Guatemalan Mayan Elders of the Eagle Clan, *The Mystery of 2012: Predictions, Prophecies and Possibilities*, Gregg Braden, others, Sounds True, 2009, p. 282.
6. Mayan Priest Carlos Barrios, *The New Humanity On The New Earth*, Hopi Newsletter Techqua Ikachi, August 30, 2008, with permission from Bill Tenuto.

Healing

Epigraph: Borysenko, Joan, *Healers on Healing*, Edited by Richard Carlson, PhD, and Benjamin Shield, Jeremy P. Tarcher, Inc. 1989, p. 189.

1. The Buddha, *Success Consciousness*, www.successconsciousness. com

2. Brooke Medicine Eagle, *Healers on Healing*, Edited by Richard Carlson, PhD, and Benjamin Shield, Jeremy P. Tarcher, Inc. 1989, p. 189.

3. _____. Armstrong, Karen, *The Reason of Faith*, *Ode Magazine*, September / October 2009, p. 38.

4. _____. 17th Karmapa, *Kindness Is the Most Important Thing*, *Shambhala Sun*, September 2008, p. 70.

Lighten Up

Epigraph: White, E.B., *The Winners Manual: For the Game of Life*. By Jim Tressel, John Maxwell, Chris Fabry, Contributor John Maxwell, Chris Fabry. Published by Tyndale House Publishers, Inc., 2008, p. 41.

1. Kataria, Dr. Madan, *Enlighten up!* Movie by Kate Churchill, with New York journalist Nick Rosen, 2008.

2. The Buddha, *1,001 Pearls of YogaWisdom: Take Your Practice Beyond the Mat.*, By Liz Lark, Duncan Baird Publishers, 2008, p, 163.

The author wishes to thank and acknowledge those who he was unable to find or gather permission to reprint their material. If the copyright holder wishes to contact the publisher or author regarding use herein of its material, the publisher will use every effort to ensure that proper credit will appear when appropriate in all future editions of this book. Namaste.

QUICK ORDER FORM

Website Orders: Please go to www.Holmanhealthconnections.com and follow the book order links.

Telephone Orders: Call 425-303-8150. Have credit card ready (or leave message and we will call you back soon).

Postal Orders: Send check to Holman Health Connections, 1917 Rockefeller Ave., Everett, WA 98201 USA

Name: _____

Address: _____ State: _____ Zip: _____

Phone: _____

Email (to receive Roy's Enewsletter): _____

Please send me _____ (quantity) of Healing Self, Healing Earth,
knowing that I may return them for full refund within 30 days.

Books _____ @ $15.95 each =   _____

Shipping: $4.00 for first book, and $2.00 for each additional book: _____

International: $8.00 for first book, and $4.00 each additional book: _____

Sales Tax: WA state residents please add appropriate sales tax: _____

Total enclosed: _____

Thank you!

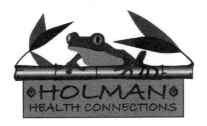

QUICK ORDER FORM

Website Orders: Please go to www.Holmanhealthconnections.com and follow the book order links.

Telephone Orders: Call 425-303-8150. Have credit card ready (or leave message and we will call you back soon).

Postal Orders: Send check to Holman Health Connections, 1917 Rockefeller Ave., Everett, WA 98201 USA

Name: _____

Address: _____ State: _____ Zip: _____

Phone: _____

Email (to receive Roy's Enewsletter): _____

Please send me _____ (quantity) of Healing Self, Healing Earth, knowing that I may return them for full refund within 30 days.

Books _____ @ $15.95 each = _____

Shipping: $4.00 for first book, and $2.00 for each additional book: _____

International: $8.00 for first book, and $4.00 each additional book: _____

Sales Tax: WA state residents please add appropriate sales tax: _____

Total enclosed: _____

Thank you!